MAKE IT HAPPEN

MAKE IT HAPPEN

Jennifer

AN INSPIRATION TO US ALL

PAUL ROBERTS

Matador
9 Priory Business Park,
Wistow Road, Kibworth Beauchamp,
Leicestershire. LE8 0RX
Tel: (+44) 116 279 2299
Fax: (+44) 116 279 2277
Email: books@troubador.co.uk
Web: www.troubador.co.uk/matador

ISBN 978 1784621 797

British Library Cataloguing in Publication Data.
A catalogue record for this book is available from the British Library.

Typeset by Troubador Publishing Ltd, Leicester, UK
Matador is an imprint of Troubador Publishing Ltd

Printed and bound in the UK by TJ International, Padstow, Cornwall

Contents

Foreword

I felt very honoured to be asked to contribute the foreword to Paul's book about Jennifer.

We knew each other for over twenty years, and dipped in and out of each other's lives as happens when you know someone for a long time.

What I saw in Jennifer was a tremendously courageous, professional and hard-working individual who was always ready to meet any challenge with tenacity, good humour and a huge reserve of spirituality.

Jennifer was often the first person I would think of when thorny questions needed a clear head, and a compassionate but no-nonsense approach.

She dealt incredibly well with all the disparate demands on her, and I never once heard her use the fact of her transplant as an excuse to be given any special treatment.

In her professional life she could deal with problem after problem and then say 'next' in a cheery voice – always willing to go the extra mile to help others.

In her personal life too she would always give of herself very generously, offering support tinged with a strong dose of reality.

Looking back on our time together, the thing I remember most is the laughter. When Jennifer was around it would always be a good day.

This book is not only a personal tribute to Jennifer from her soulmate Paul, but it is also a beacon of hope for those living life with a kidney transplant or cancer.

It is hoped that proceeds from the sale will help others to face this challenge with the fortitude and good humour with which Jennifer approached her own life.

Those who knew her personally were very privileged. Those who can know her story from this book will be able to share some of the strength and resilience which she brought to her life, and from which we can all benefit.

I hope that you enjoy this excellent tribute to Jennifer which will stand as a very fitting memorial to a really lovely person.

Lesley Rimmer OBE
Former Chief Executive of the United Kingdom
Home Care Association

1.

Our love story

Two extraordinary happenings have shaped my life – one that led to a successful twenty-six year career as a newspaper journalist, and another that resulted in me marrying one of the most remarkable women of our times.

The almost unbelievable occurrences – securing a job I was never meant to have and a highly improbable blind date with a long-term kidney transplant patient – give credence to the theory that truth is stranger than fiction.

Born in a small rural community in the heart of Devon, I had few expectations as a young man. One of six children, I grew up on a small farm on the outskirts of a remote village which had been our family home since January 1940.

At sixteen, and in my last year at Chulmleigh Community College in 1974, I thought hard about following in my dad's footsteps and embarking on a career in agriculture.

I considered the possibility of taking on Farthing Park, our thirty-six acre dairy farm near Morchard Bishop, sometime in the future, perhaps when my parents had retired.

But the prospects were not good. Dad was having to work on a neighbouring farm as well as his own to keep it going, and mum was struggling to make ends meet and to keep our large family fed and clothed.

She knew I had a strong desire to be a writer and encouraged me to follow my heart and pursue a career I wanted to have rather than one I was expected to follow. She was right, of course, and I took her advice.

I wrote to the editors of fifty different newspapers across the UK, asking them to consider taking me on as a trainee reporter. I had just one positive reply – from John Page, the then editor of *The Cornishman*.

He offered me an interview and I travelled to Penzance in Cornwall to see him in the summer of 1974. I thought it went well, but heard nothing in the following weeks.

I plucked up the courage to phone him and was told I had been shortlisted for a job. Ten days later, a letter arrived for me at my home. I opened it, fearing the worst.

It was from Mr Page and said: *Dear Roger... I would like to offer you the post of trainee reporter.* He got the name wrong, but I couldn't have been more thrilled.

Within a month I moved to Cornwall and worked hard to make my mark at the newspaper. In 1978 I was offered a promotion – as *The Cornishman's* district correspondent for St Ives, Hayle, Camborne, Redruth, Helston and Porthleven.

As Mr Page called me into his office to congratulate me on my new role, he dropped the bombshell news that he had made a 'terrible mistake' in appointing me as a trainee four years earlier, one that he had initially struggled to live with.

He told me I had not been selected for the role. Someone called Roger had secured the post, but had received the 'sorry Paul' reply intended for me. Essentially, I had got the job because I received the wrong letter.

Mr Page, seeing my head drop into my hands in despair, quickly assured me that I had proved him wrong. I turned out to be the 'right choice' and had made the most of an opportunity which should never have come my way.

I never looked back. After ten very happy years at *The Cornishman*, I left to become a reporter for *The West Briton*, Cornwall's largest selling weekly newspaper, working my way up to eventually become its editor.

In 1995, I led the transformation of the paper from a broadsheet to a tabloid format, helping it to win Britain's weekly newspaper of the year award and to become the bestselling paid-for weekly in the UK.

I later became assistant editor of *The Western Morning News* and publisher and launch editor of a new quality magazine, *Devon Today*, my final role as a journalist after a career with the Harmsworth Group.

My job was my hobby and my hobby was my job. Consequently, I was married to it for most of those years, regularly working twelve to fourteen-hour days and six-day weeks. Then, my life changed again, completely out of the blue.

I was recovering from the break-up of a twenty-year relationship – a marriage in which I had hardly seen my two children grow up because of my career – when I met Jennifer Roberts on a blind date.

It marked the start of an incredible love story and the dawn of an idyllic and hugely rewarding life with the most inspirational woman I have ever encountered.

Jennifer's story deserves to be told, hence this biography. It is called *Make it Happen* because Jennifer had the knack of making good things happen time and time again.

Those three short words formed the welcoming message on her purple mobile phone, the opening line in her diaries and notebooks, and became her business motto.

The biography focuses particularly on the years we spent together and my experience of Jennifer's achievements and positive attitude in the face of great adversity.

Paul Roberts

Two pebbles, two hearts
— how we met

The ice-cold blue waters off Iona stretched out before me as I sat on a beach on the idyllic Scottish island in early January 2001. It was cold but dry, the sun was shining as gulls screeched overhead, and I was very much alone.

I had taken a short break at an island hotel to get away from the pressures of work and had spent hours on those white sands, watching the tide and skies change and contemplating what the future would hold for me.

As I watched a small fishing boat head out to deeper waters beyond Fionnphort on the neighbouring island of Mull, I randomly picked up a small rounded pebble and threw it into the swirling sea.

In that very moment – as I was silently wishing to meet someone who would transform my life, make me happy and love me as much as I would love her – the sun shone so brightly it could have been a summer's day.

More than five hundred miles away, on the same day, Jennifer threw a pebble into the sea from the windswept sands at Burnham-on-Sea, Somerset. It was cast into the waters with the same wishes, the same hopes.

At the time I was a magazine publisher and editor after working for regional newspapers for twenty-five years. I was tired of the job, my health was suffering and I was receiving medical treatment for high blood pressure.

I had taken the New Year break in Iona because, at the age of forty-two, I was at a crossroads in my life. I was trying to work out whether I needed a career change and how I could find some happiness.

Minutes after watching my pebble disappear into the ocean, after skipping three times along the surface, I walked to Iona Abbey and sat in silence in one of Scotland's oldest, most sacred and historic buildings for more than two hours.

These were defining moments for me. For the first time in many months I experienced peace and calm in this spiritual haven, and found the will and determination to do everything I could to turn my life round.

On my return to my then coastal home in Instow, in North Devon, I decided to try and meet someone through a mobile phone dating service which published details of people 'looking for love' in a 'lonely hearts' column in my local newspaper.

I was totally unaware that my appeal for a partner would appear in many different publications throughout the South West of England – including Jennifer's local weekly newspaper, the *Burnham and Highbridge Gazette*.

There was no reason for Jennifer to be looking in the *Gazette* for a new man in her life. She was trying to find a 'life partner' through a professional dating agency and had been given a list of potential suitors 'fitting her profile'.

But late one Saturday night she saw my words by pure chance as she was about to throw the newspaper away. She was dropping it into a rubbish bin when she came across the lonely hearts page, and liked what I had to say.

She didn't call me straight away. She was nervous about meeting a 'complete stranger' through a newspaper column. A friend with her at the time encouraged her to make contact – and she left a message for me.

I was away at the time, in Stirling, visiting its formidable castle and touring Scotland's lochs and glens. I never imagined anyone would respond to my lonely hearts plea. I genuinely thought I had made a fool of myself in making it.

When I returned home a week later, I picked up Jennifer's message. It was so cheery, so inviting, and so warm, I didn't hesitate in calling her. I immediately apologised for taking so long to get back to her and she instantly accepted my explanation.

We talked for hours on the phone in the five days before meeting for the first time at the less than romantic Exeter Services Station in Devon on January 27, 2001, arriving in the car park there in separate cars.

As I walked towards Jennifer's blue Hyundai Coupe, she opened the door and put her right hand out for a welcoming handshake. I took her long and delicate fingers in mine and gave her a warm kiss on the cheek.

She was a little surprised by my eagerness, to the point where she forgot to put the handbrake on her car as she was getting out of it. It rolled down the car park for a few yards before she was able to stop it moving, with me standing behind it clinging on to the boot.

I thought I had blown my chances with her before our date had even got off the ground. But she agreed to share a meal with me at one of my favourite pubs, the picturesque, thatched Blue Ball Inn at nearby Topsham.

As I ordered our first drinks, Jennifer said she had to go to the ladies. I instantly thought she was going to phone a friend to come and 'rescue' her, or would return with an excuse that she couldn't stay because 'something had turned up'.

How wrong I was. She explained that a slip under her dress had started to fall down and she had to carry out 'urgent repairs'. I joked about my fears. Jennifer said she had phoned a friend... but only to say she was really looking forward to our date.

As we sat and talked, we made an instant connection. I liked the way she looked, warmed to her amazing smile and loved hearing about her work – she was then co-owner of a sound wave therapy business – and interests.

We could hardly believe that we had thrown pebbles into the sea at opposite ends of the UK just twenty-two days earlier. It seemed that fate had intervened to bring us together, and we both seemed fully aware of the significance of it all.

We fell in love almost at first sight, connecting in every way within the first hour of our meeting. I can't explain it, but I knew on that first date that we would spend the rest of our lives together.

We talked and talked, well past closing time when we were the last ones in the Blue Ball, not wanting the evening to end. We ended up back at Exeter Services, to enjoy midnight coffees and more chat.

We kissed each other passionately before going our separate ways. We talked again the next day and were inseparable by the following weekend. Within a few weeks we were living together and planning the rest of our lives.

We lived at Burnham-on-Sea. By then I had left my work as a publisher and editor and took temporary employment locally as a touring site warden and security guard at a local holiday park, while Jennifer continued her sound wave therapy business.

Jennifer was proud that I had been prepared to take work at

£4 an hour after leaving a demanding career that paid me £50,000+ a year. I enjoyed a nine to five job after the stress-filled eighty-hour weeks I had been used to.

The holiday park work produced almost as much drama as a busy day in a newspaper office. There were daily mishaps from an expensive new caravan being wrecked while crashing through manhole covers to poorly erected fences collapsing minutes after being put up.

My little HQ for welcoming touring vans – a tiny caravan that could not be locked – was gradually dismantled by thieves. Seats, doors, fabric, clothes and my desk were stolen over a period of weeks, leaving me with just a shell to operate from.

I almost caught fire while operating a sit-down lawn mower that burst into flames. I shouted 'fire' to my boss on my two-way radio. He and three colleagues came running armed with fire extinguishers, but it was too late to save the mower.

Nine months after we met, and just over seventeen years after Jennifer had had a kidney transplant, we became engaged at a party attended by family and friends at the Battleborough Grange Hotel near Burnham-on-Sea.

The party, a 'celebration of life, love and new beginnings', was full of surprises. The greatest of which was Jennifer falling to one knee and proposing to me in front of a large audience – just as I thought I would be doing the honours.

We holidayed in Paris and then started the next chapter of our journey together – buying and running a very busy fish and chip takeaway and restaurant in a beautiful coastal village in Dorset.

In March 2003, we were married at Dundas Castle at South Queensferry, near Edinburgh. The remarkable story of how we met was told by me at the ceremony in my poem – *Two pebbles, two hearts... our love story.*

The still blue waters of Iona swallowed up the tiny pebble,
Thrown by a lonely figure looking out to sea,
It carried with it all his hopes...
For true love, a new life – to be as happy as a man can be.
The wishes seemed so distant... the impossible dream.
Even on this magical island, so peaceful, so serene.
But as the sun shone brightly on the glistening white sands,
The impossible was about to happen for this enlightened man.

Five hundred miles away on a windswept Somerset beach,
A beautiful woman cast another pebble into the ocean deep.
She shared the same desire for love, happiness, a new beginning.
The little stone represented all those hopes, a symbol of her craving.
The seeds were sown for a remarkable love.
So pure, so real, forever burning bright.
Two hearts merging as one,
Now ready to set the world alight.
Romance blossomed at the dawn of a new year.
Fate uniting two people in the wake of festive cheer.
Togetherness sealed through a 'lonely hearts' plea.
A love akin to a sacred flame, destined to burn eternally.

I recited the poem eighteen days later when a special service of blessing was held at our parish church in Charmouth in Dorset. I read it ten years later when we celebrated our tenth wedding anniversary, renewed our vows and exchanged more rings in a private villa in Playa Blanca on Lanzarote in the Canary Islands.

And it was read again on November 22, 2013, at St Mary's Church, Aberfoyle, this time by Rector Richard Grosse at the service to celebrate the life of Jennifer – thirteen days after she passed away at the Forth Valley Royal Hospital in Larbert, Stirlingshire.

A March wedding in Scotland – you must be mad

Some thought we were mad. 'A March wedding... in Scotland! You'll be lucky to get there through the snow,' one friend told us. But the date and venue were fixed and Jennifer assured everyone, including me, that the sun would shine on us on our big day.

It did, in a record-breaking way. Our wedding took place as Scotland enjoyed its hottest March for forty-two years in 2003. *The Scotsman* reported that temperatures soared to nineteen degrees centigrade in the sunniest and driest March since 1961.

It was the icing on the cake for a genuine fairy tale wedding at an authentic Scottish castle near Edinburgh. But it could have been so different if, as originally planned, we had married there six months earlier.

Storms, with gale force winds and torrential rain, battered the UK in October 2002, halting rail and air services, bringing trees crashing down from Cornwall to the far north of Scotland, leaving a trail of wreckage in its wake.

We had delayed our wedding because of work commitments at our new takeaway and restaurant business, and because Jennifer was convinced that the weather would be 'too challenging' at that time of the year.

Why get married in Scotland? Well, I succumbed to its mountains, lochs and wide open spaces on visits many years before. And it was where my quest for a life partner and kindred spirit had begun.

Jennifer fell in love with Scotland as much as me as we holidayed there in our early days together. She truly believed it was our 'spiritual home' and was convinced that, eventually, we would make our home there.

Our wedding took place at the fifteenth century Auld Keep at Dundas Castle at South Queensferry, near Edinburgh, built by the renowned architect William Burn, and home to the Stewart-Clark family since the late 1800s.

We orchestrated the entire event with the help of Dundas staff – from the music, words and vows for the ceremony to the wedding breakfast, flowers and the ceilidh that rounded off a truly perfect day.

Jennifer chose beautiful choral pieces from Libera and the mesmeric 'All Love Can Be' from the film *A Beautiful Mind* for the wedding itself. She entered the Auld Keep to the atmospheric music of *Braveheart*, so appropriate for my courageous wife.

Before the wedding breakfast, Jennifer and I and all our eighteen guests drank whisky from a Scottish Quaich we had bought from the famous Luckenbooth shop on Edinburgh's Royal Mile and quoted verse written by poet Robert Burns.

We had use of the castle for two days, holding a pre-wedding party in the Stag Room there the night before. Our first day as bride and groom was spent in an idyllic boat house on a private loch in the castle grounds.

It was the most memorable time of our lives, spent with family and friends who had supported and encouraged us. It was also a celebration so richly deserved by Jennifer, who had devoted her life to helping others.

The significance of it all is summed up in letters Jennifer and I exchanged in the hours leading up to the wedding ceremony, as we reflected on the incredible series of events that had brought us together to fall so much in love.

Jennifer wrote:

> *Today is the day that I have dreamed about all of my life. To marry a man who loves me as much as I love him. Who thinks about me, my needs, hopes and dreams. A man who cares for me in every way, every day.*
>
> *The timepiece I give to you today (a Dalvey pocket watch) is symbolic in so many ways. It comes from Scotland where our hearts will be joined forever. It symbolises the most precious gift that you can give anyone and that is your time. Time to listen, time to speak, time to love, time to care, time to dream, time to support, time to laugh.*
>
> *I dreamed for you, prayed for you, yearned for you. I have to pinch myself to believe that you are here in the flesh and that you love me as much as I love you. My greatest achievement will be to marry you and continue to make you happy for the rest of your life.*

I wrote:

> *We met twenty-seven months ago on a blind date. We have lived life to the full, shared every up and down imaginable and become soulmates, lovers, friends, companions and partners. Today is the fulfilment of all*

our dreams – to marry the perfect partner in the perfect location.

We have both waited so long for this moment. To see it coming to fruition today is a real-life miracle. Ours is the greatest fairy tale wedding imaginable.

Planning our wedding was not all plain sailing. A month before our big day, we arranged to drive to Edinburgh from Charmouth in Dorset to visit the wedding caterers to sample the food we had chosen.

When we got to Carlisle, the M6 was hit by a blizzard which brought much of the traffic to a standstill. I, perhaps stupidly, decided to head on to Edinburgh in the wake of lorries bulldozing their way through the snow.

I was driving a Mitsubishi Space Star, hardly equipped for the conditions, but somehow I managed to keep going for the next one hundred miles, negotiating multiple diversions and weaving in and out of abandoned vehicles on the motorway and A roads.

Jennifer sat nervously in the front passenger seat, armed with a map and torch to help get us to our destination. We both knew we were lucky to get to the Scottish capital in one piece, particularly as roads became indistinguishable in the constantly falling snow.

When we first looked at wedding venues in 2002, Scotland was hit by some of the worst storms for many years. Roofs were blown off homes, and industrial buildings and hundreds of trees were brought down by hurricane force winds during our visit.

We were staying at a hotel on Loch Lomond when Jennifer's mum made a desperate call to us asking us if we had seen the devastation on the TV, and very much hoping that we were okay. We were oblivious to what was going on around us.

At one stage I asked Jennifer if she would prefer to get married further south. She just looked at me, smiled and said: 'Of course not. Scotland is where we want to get married and we will. The weather can't be like this all the time.'

Our wedding was notable for two key events – the record-breaking March temperatures and the invasion of Iraq by America, Britain and other international forces in a conflict that later became known as the Iraq War.

The day of our wedding was also the 697th anniversary of Robert the Bruce being chosen as King of the Scots. He was crowned two days later to lead the fight for Scottish independence against King Edward I of England.

We honeymooned in Scotland's little known Ardnamurchan peninsula, staying in a remarkable romantic and eccentric circular folly, the Tower at Greenwood, overlooking Loch Sunart, before heading to Iona.

We stayed at the island's nineteenth century Argyll Hotel, near the beach where more than two years earlier I had wished to find someone as lovely as Jennifer as I threw that small, round grey pebble into the sea.

The fine weather continued for the whole of our honeymoon. It was so hot we both got sunburnt on the island's white sands. We knew we had been blessed in so many ways. The sun had smiled on us and our burgeoning relationship.

More than one hundred people later attended our marriage blessing at St Andrew's Parish Church, Charmouth. Again, it was another hot, beautiful day.

A marriage made in heaven

It's easy to dismiss the romantics and poets who eulogise about finding the perfect love and sharing life with a 'soulmate' or 'kindred spirit'. For many, it is the stuff of fantasy, something that never happens to us.

You only have to browse through lonely hearts columns in newspapers and online to discover how many people are searching – very often fruitlessly – for a lasting, loving relationship which will change their lives for the good.

I remember as a young newspaper reporter seeing moving death notices for the young and old reflecting on the loss of not only a dear wife or husband, but a 'spiritual twin', 'twin flame', 'twin heart', 'everything that's good in my life'.

I often wondered what it was like to be in such a relationship, to be totally immersed in the life of another, to love and be loved in equal measure. I found out after I met Jennifer on our blind date.

Within days we could barely stand being away from each other. Our lives were intertwining so fast. Living more than one hundred miles apart at that stage, we talked endlessly on the phone until we could meet again.

In less than a week we were inseparable, sending each other beautifully worded cards and letters almost on a daily basis, expressing our undying love for each other. It was extraordinary but it seemed perfectly natural.

Inside two months we were living together at Jennifer's home in Burnham-on-Sea, planning our engagement and wedding, and looking at starting or taking on a business that would bring us even closer.

We took a leap into the unknown when we purchased the fish bar and restaurant in Charmouth, near Lyme Regis, a village renowned for its fossil beach and which became part of a World Heritage Site shortly after our arrival.

It was a daunting challenge for us – a journalist who couldn't cook and a nurse with limited experience in catering – and one that would have taxed even the most experienced and devoted of couples.

But we took it in our stride thanks to Jennifer's amazing belief in me and in us. Long days, extremely hard work and the occasional difficult customer didn't faze us. Jennifer always said that, together, we could and would achieve great things. And she was right.

We worked so well as a team. We knew instinctively what we needed and when, never stopped smiling even when things were going wrong and our love for each other continued to grow in the toughest of work environments.

We took time to write cards and letters to each other, very often after midnight when the chippy had closed, regularly exchanged gifts and talked encouragingly about the day ahead, even when we were exhausted.

We closed the chippy for birthdays and anniversaries, even in busy times, because of our firm belief that we should put ourselves first and not allow the business to become more important than our private lives.

We took that philosophy to Scotland when we moved there six years later. We bought a house in a tranquil and remote area of the Trossachs, on the banks of Loch Katrine, hardly believing our good fortune to be moving to such a beautiful area.

We wanted to escape the 'rat race', to enjoy life in one of the quietest and most secluded areas of Britain. We also wanted to take our relationship to a new level – spending all our time together, with hardly a minute apart.

Within the next twelve months, Jennifer started a new business, a consultancy specialising in home care and dementia, that would enable us to work together, and from home, and give us the work-life balance we were looking for.

The move, the business, and our never flagging excitement at being in the heart of Scotland, helped us to achieve all we were looking for and much more. Our unbreakable relationship became ever stronger, our love for each other reaching new heights.

We did all the things we promised we would – holidaying in virtually every corner and nook of mainland Scotland and its many isles, creating a beautiful spiritual garden outside our home and spending more quality time together.

When I was a cub reporter on *The Cornishman* newspaper in Penzance, I very often met and wrote about couples celebrating great milestones in their lives – golden, diamond or platinum wedding anniversaries.

One of the questions I would always ask those lucky couples was the secret of their marital success. Many would say being able to 'give and take', to listen to each other, to be kind and considerate and to keep smiling.

Strangely, very few ever mentioned the word love or its importance to them. Some said their marriage had survived because they spent so little time together they didn't have time to 'get on each other's nerves'!

But the couple I remember the most were a husband and wife from Carbis Bay near St Ives who were celebrating their golden wedding. When I visited their home, they were sitting on the sofa together, holding hands and looking so happy.

They were both so much in love, thrilled to be in each other's company and to have been so fortunate to have spent more than fifty years together. They kissed and hugged each other several times while I talked to them about their marriage.

The wife said the secret of their success was falling deeply in love at first sight and never wanting to be apart. They had never spent a night away from each other since they had married, and their love was as strong now as when they first met.

The husband said that each time he gazed at his wife it was as if he was looking at her for the first time. He loved her more than anyone could ever know, and he could not imagine living even a day without her.

In my years as a trainee reporter, I had the privilege to live with a loving, friendly couple and their family in Crowlas, near Penzance. Joe and Muriel Laity were totally devoted to one another, so happy in each other's company.

In all their years of marriage they were kind to each other, never argued and were openly affectionate. It was a joy to be with them and to witness how close a husband and wife could be.

I felt that what Joe and Muriel and the couple from Carbis Bay had in common was a rare and beautiful bond, seemingly unattainable for the vast majority of us, including me.

How wrong I was. I had to wait forty-two years for Jennifer to come along, but the wait was so worth it. We lived for each other and loved every minute we spent together. We were a mirror image of that couple I met in Cornwall in the 1970s, always holding hands, always hugging and kissing each other and so grateful that we had had the opportunity to share an amazing life together.

We both had no doubt that fate had brought us together when we cast those pebbles into the sea 500 miles apart shortly before we met. There may be no scientific explanation for it, but we were simply meant to be.

We were a formidable team, in our private lives and in business. We were kind and respectful to each other, but most of all we loved each other with a passion that few could ever match.

Without being in any way arrogant or dismissive of other relationships, Jennifer would often say that many people spent their whole lives looking for a little of what we had. We never took for granted how lucky we were.

On the mantelpiece of our home, there is a picture of us from our engagement party in Somerset in 2001. It's in a frame that carries the words *two hearts as one... having lots of fun*. Those eight words sum up our life perfectly.

In the many cards sent to me by Jennifer over the years, she often referred to how we had 'merged as one', physically, mentally and spiritually. Anyone knowing us, family or friends, would have agreed with that 100%.

When I was asked what Jennifer's love had done for me, I would say she had completely transformed my life – from a cynical workaholic journalist who had devoted his life to the regional newspaper industry, to a man who had truly found happiness.

I would frequently quote Jack Nicholson from the Oscar winning movie *As Good as it Gets* – particularly in a speech after my marriage – that Jennifer had made me want to be a better (and kinder) man.

Jennifer, who would tell anyone who asked that I had made

her happier than she could ever have imagined, would respond by saying that I had always been a good man but she had 'turned up the volume a little bit'.

Jennifer had just one regret; that we didn't find each other sooner so we could have loved each other for longer.

We had fewer than thirteen years together before she passed away.

But, boy, what amazing years they were.

No ordinary love

Ours was no ordinary love. We lived and worked together in complete harmony. We were in tune in every way imaginable from liking the same things to having the same interests. We never liked being apart and truly treasured every moment we shared.

In all, we spent twelve years nine months and thirteen days together. That's a total of 667 weeks, or 4,669 days, or 112,056 hours, or 403,401,600 seconds. We made every hour count and exchanged more than 1,000 love letters, cards and notes, all written with a passion and honesty that many people never experience.

On my desk, I keep a very special card given to me by Jennifer on our sixth wedding anniversary. The words in it include the following: *In you, I have found true and lasting happiness. You have made all my dreams come true... and I am proud and honoured to call myself your wife.*

In finding you, my soulmate, it feels that my life only really started when you came into it. Our love is like the brightest beacon on earth, the richest oasis in the driest desert, a paradise like no other. We are so lucky to have each other, so fortunate to have met when we did. Life is just wonderful with you.

Those eighty-nine words of the thousands we wrote to each other encapsulate our rare and special love. The following extracts from our cards and letters give an insight into the depth of our feelings for each other from when we first met in January 2001, and the extraordinary woman I married.

Card from Jennifer marking the ninth anniversary of our first date

Many things happened in my life before you came. One very vivid recollection was standing on a beach in Burnham-on-Sea and asking why wasn't there someone for me. I then felt moved to pick up a pebble and dared to wish, dream for my perfect partner. I thought long and hard about this dream person and then I kissed the pebble and threw it with all my hopes and dreams into the sea. January is traditionally a month of bland following the Christmas celebrations. But this January was a once in a lifetime month, my wish, dreams and prayers were answered. My darling Paul arrived in my life and everything fell into place. We have endured many difficult times together, but these have been overshadowed by an amazing love, trust, friendship and a deep spiritual understanding and commitment. My life is completely entwined with yours. I feel like my heart beats when yours does, our very breath and pulse move seamlessly together. It is a harmony that can't be grown or created. It is a natural rhythm that exists between the two of us. This is a special day – it's the day God put you in my way.

Card from me, written after midnight on February 21, 2001

Just over a month ago I sat on a pretty little beach on Iona, resting place of Scotland's ancient kings, looking out to sea – and wondering what the future would bring. As I basked in the sunshine I made a wish that I would meet someone who would love me as much as I would love her. At that time, it seemed such a remote possibility. I had so much love to give, but had failed to find my soulmate in forty-two years. Yet, the spiritual strength I gained on Iona gave me new hope. I knew there was someone out there for me – someone who would want me as much as I wanted her. When I first met you, I had this feeling that there was something very special happening. My wish, declared on Iona, came sharply into focus in the following two weeks as we grew closer. My dream, my wish, has come true thanks to you.

Jennifer's wedding anniversary card to Paul, 2004

If you see half the love that you give me reflected back in my eyes... you would be blinded by the light. You are the part of me that allows my soul to soar and my spirit to sing. My strength, my belief, my hope and passion stems like a fountain out of a Scottish spring constantly fed and tended by your love for me.

Card from me, sent March 6, 2001

It's remarkable how one thing – a stroke of luck, perhaps, or fate playing its hand – can change your life. When I was sixteen I left school with little prospect of carving out a career for myself. A life in farming beckoned. I was the eldest son on my dad's farm and expected to succeed him. That was exactly what I didn't want. I knew there was no future in farming on a smallholding sandwiched between two giant farms. I had ambitions to be a writer and ended up getting a job on a weekly newspaper that I should never have had. My application for a trainee reporter's role was turned down but, amazingly, I received the letter intended for the person who was successful. Strange, but true. And something which shaped my whole career. More than twenty-six years later, another remarkable series of circumstances led to you and I meeting at the Blue Ball, Exeter. I signed up with a mobile dating agency – something I thought I would never do. I went away for a week, during which you contacted me. I almost missed your message and thought you may have found someone else by the time we made contact. But we talked... and talked. And when we met it was as if I had been waiting for that very moment. The words meant to be were stamped all over our first date. We have never looked back. There were all sorts of reasons why we were not going to meet up – you could have missed my ad, you could have been seeing someone else at the time. I could have missed your message. But fate played its hand. We were meant to meet on January 27, 2001. What a wonderful beginning.

Jennifer's Christmas card to me, 2011

My greatest gift, I give to you, is the one that is only shared by you and me. My life, work, happiness and health are wholly sustained by you. The gift I give you is to love and support you every day. My gift is love, pure and simple, unconditional and wrapped up with faith and tied up with ribbons of hope, expectation, excitement and the knowledge that anything you want to achieve is possible. This special gift is not just for Christmas, this gift is there for you every day of the year for the rest of our lives. I did not think it was possible to feel such love, affection and adoration for another person and sometimes those feelings *are scary – but only because of the fear of the time when we will part.*

Christmas card from me, 2004

In my weakest moments you are always there. When I need love and affection you are always there. When I need a cuddle and a friendly chat you are always there.

Christmas card from Jennifer, 2009

Behind every great woman there is an incredible man, and I am truly blessed that I have you. You have given me everything I could ever need. You see before me what I need and you give it so lovingly; many things every day that help me in life. Without you I would be a pale shadow, slipping past people unnoticed. With you I shine, grow and am able to be truly me. With you I can achieve anything. Thank you, my darling for finding me, marrying me and sharing my every step. I am yours today, tomorrow, and forever. Our spirits are truly joined for eternity.

Birthday card from me, 2009

I feel as if our years together are like an ever improving wine... gaining in value, maturity and importance. Every day is like sipping the finest Bordeaux – a rich elixir of love, affection and beautiful friendship.

Christmas card from Jennifer, 2007

Sometimes I ask myself what it is about us that makes what we have so magical. Is it that we have been together through some difficult times? Is it because we have the same interests? Perhaps it's because we share our work, drive and passion for making a difference together. Maybe it's because we live in the most amazing place, where sheer beauty inspires us. It could be that we are comfortable in the silence of being together. But on top of all this I believe it's because we are joined at a deep spiritual, pure love level. I see you... and you see me and we both reflect that love, admiration and respect. Our love is deep and true and nothing will shake it. We will stay together and into eternity. A love that shines so bright it's dazzling.

Letter from me, September 2001

How do I love thee? With all the passion of a Mozart opera and a Tchaikovsky symphony. With the gentle romance of a Rachmaninov overture and stirring emotion of a Beethoven concerto.

Wedding anniversary card from Jennifer, 2008

Seven years ago I could never have imagined the journey I was about to take. We have overcome so many things. We have enjoyed the good times and had moments when words could not describe the love and understanding we have reached. A unique partnership that few could understand. Our life in Scotland could not be better. The place we live is beyond my wildest dreams and the love and joy of life we have found here is indescribable.

Birthday card from me, 2007

It's your first birthday in Scotland, the country that has become our home, our sanctuary, the hub of our daily lives and dreams. In just a few short days we will have been in Stronachlachar for six months. For all the right reasons, it feels as if we have been here for years. I don't think we have ever been happier. Days come and go, the seasons change, the weather brings new surprises every week. But our love for this place never diminishes. Our journey here is a remarkable tale, but just another chapter in our extraordinary lives together. Many would never believe how we ended up here. Let alone how we met and faced so many challenges together. Sometimes it feels almost beyond belief what we have achieved together.

Christmas card from Jennifer, 2007

A year ago it would have been impossible to imagine ourselves here in Scotland, in a beautiful cottage surrounded by the most amazing countryside. I am so happy and content here it would be difficult to put it into words. Just like my love for you, it grows through the seasons, shining brightly in the summer and keeping me warm in the winter. It's as steady and deep as the lochs and as tall and majestic as the mountains, and it will stretch into the universe like the stars.

Valentine's card from Jennifer, 2002

From the moment I met you I wanted to proclaim my love for you from the rooftops. My love for you is like a raindrop in a stream – it started as a little ripple and then grew to such intensity that it would now fill an ocean. From space you could see the energy that my love for you generates. It would eclipse the earth.

Birthday card from me, 2011

Love can't be measured, it doesn't grow on trees, you can't touch it. But when you are with the right person you can see it every day, experience the excitement it brings, feel the warmth it brings. We are so lucky that we can share in the exhilaration all these emotions deliver. The tenderness, the good times we share are so precious. We are as one in almost everything we do. Two people could not be closer, could not love each other more. It is so rare to find a couple who live and work together, who work and exist as one unit, who totally adore each other.

Christmas card from me, 2012

Being with you and enjoying every minute we have together is the greatest gift anyone could give me. Your life has been remarkable in so many ways. You treat adversity and triumph in the same way. You always look for the best in people. You bring out the best in everyone, including me. These are qualities that are so rare.

Birthday card from Jennifer, 2006

My gift to you is eternal love beyond the bounds of everyday imagination – a cup of love always full, only for you.

Wedding anniversary card from Jennifer, 2013

We had the hottest week on record for our honeymoon in Scotland. We should have known that this would be a sign to mark our whole life... always surprising, always turning out for the best. During our ten years we have achieved so much in our lives. Our journey has brought us successful businesses. We have enjoyed many amazing holidays. Both Pauls I described on my wedding day – the Paul everyone knew and the private Paul I get to see – have been present every step of the way, never faltering, never changing, a unique and constant blend that enables me to be surefooted every day.

Most recently we have been challenged with a health issue. At this point I have never known such strength, such belief, such love, such confidence in any man. My darling Paul stood tall, my rock which carries me on. Today will be emotional... but above all our love will be so bright, so strong, and so deep it will rock the world.

Letter from Jennifer with Jack Vettriano's 'Singing Butler' on the front, 2006 (during poor health in our last summer at the takeaway in Charmouth)

I feel the picture reflects how I am feeling. Storms all around me, but the one thing that I know for sure is that there are two elegant, beautiful people dancing in the centre that are us. No matter what life dishes up for us, I know that we will hang on to true love and friendship for eternity. I have wished for you all my life and you have not been a disappointment in any way.

Card from me marking the tenth anniversary of our first date, 2011

How time flies. Ten years ago today I met this beautiful woman in a car park near Exeter, dined with her at the Blue Ball Inn, Topsham, and enjoyed frothy coffee at a service station. How could I have known then that this gorgeous woman would become my wife, my best friend, my soulmate, my inspiration? But in many ways I did. I fell in love with you almost at first glance. That wonderful evening together in January 2001 was the beginning of something remarkable, rare and beautiful. Ten years on, I still look at you as if I was meeting you for the first time. I love you more than ever. You are everything I could ever have hoped for. And more.

Wedding anniversary card from me, 2013

How do you sum up in words an amazing journey that began on January 27, 2001 and led to the happiest day of my life on March 25, 2003 – the day you became my wife? The greatest library on earth, holding all the books ever published, could not do justice to the depth of love and feeling I have for you. There are not enough words in the English language to describe how much I adore you. There are not enough hours in a day, or days in a year to tell you how much you mean to me. For me, our wedding was the greatest day of my life – and the beginning of a new symphony of love, togetherness and affection that few will ever match.

Birthday card from me, 2010

Our love has grown beyond comparison. Our lives are intertwined in a way many would find unfathomable.

Wedding anniversary card from Jennifer, 2007

You have made my life complete. You have provided so many amazing memories and experiences. And through all the years your love has wound its way through like a beautiful thread in a perfect tapestry.

Birthday card from Jennifer, 2013

Paul is the man who makes me laugh every day... a rare gift. Paul is practical... he looks after our home, making it warm, cosy and beautiful just for me. Paul arranges lovely breaks and holidays but very much with me in mind. Paul is the most loyal, amazing friend you could ever wish to have. Paul is my business partner, protecting me like a tiger – always looking after my best *interests. The quiet man behind me all the way. Paul is my lover, gentle, caring, compassionate and deeply moving. Paul has a deep strength and wisdom often overlooked but never forgotten. The day you were born was very important for a number of reasons, particularly for your dear mum, dad and family. But for me, it was the first day you started working towards me – and that, more than anything, is worth celebrating today and every year.*

The chip shop years — our venture into the unknown

The queue seemed endless. The temperature was soaring to over one hundred degrees Fahrenheit, and we had never worked so hard in all our lives. The summer holidays had just begun, marking the start of forty-two non-stop fifteen-hour days of relentless, yet rewarding, toil.

We would each drink up to eight pints of water as we cooked and served hundreds of meals in five hours of evening bliss and madness. Laughter, good banter, praise from customers and a good night's takings were remuneration for the most exhausting rollercoaster 'ride' in the world of catering.

Only those who have worked in a very busy fish and chip takeaway can really understand the exacting nature of the work – and the toll it can take.

Jennifer and I ran the fish and chip takeaway in Charmouth for five years, a business we were both told that we could and should not operate.

Although Jennifer had previously worked behind the bar in

pubs and clubs, neither of us had ever run a catering business before.

We knew nothing about fish and chips, apart from liking them. We were given a day's tuition on battering cod and making chips by the previous owners and were then left to get on with it.

It was decided that I would become the fryer because of the physical challenge it presented. It was perhaps overlooked that I had never cooked before in my life.

Not surprisingly, some friends – and people concerned for Jennifer's health and wellbeing – suggested it was a step too far for us.

But we liked being thrown in the deep end... to have the chance to prove the doubters wrong. For Jennifer it was another opportunity to defy the odds.

The truth is we were both ready for a new challenge. My career in newspapers was over and Jennifer needed a break from her care consultancy work.

Most importantly, we both wanted to work together and try something new in a beautiful area that we both loved.

Fortunately, we had a gentle introduction to life in the chippy, taking it over in the quiet winter months.

It gave us time to 'bed in' and build up our catering and front-of-house skills before the onset of Easter and out first summer season.

Nothing really prepared us for the huge surge in business. The constant queues of customers and 'cooking to order' hundreds of meals a day were frequently a formidable challenge.

But we came through it with great aplomb, nearly always enjoying the work and making many friends along the way.

Jennifer's stamina, grit, dedication, organisational skills and tremendous will to succeed never ceased to amaze me.

She was a brilliant front-of-house operator, always smiling, always cracking jokes – keeping long queues of customers entertained as they waited for their food.

In five successful years we transformed the chippy from a seasonal to an all-year-round business, doubling the turnover.

Our time there culminated in us winning a *Good Eating Guide* certificate of outstanding achievement for 'consistently maintaining very high standards of traditional quality and customer service'.

Jennifer was a great all-rounder, turning her hand to any task that needed doing – from serving customers and cleaning to looking after the accounts and health and safety work.

She ran the business almost single-handedly when I was rushed to hospital after collapsing in the chippy with kidney stones.

She not only kept the takeaway open on a day-to-day basis during that period, but also found time to visit me at Dorchester Hospital.

She never panicked when things went wrong, particularly when we were hit by power cuts and when the fryers, so vital to our business, were out of action.

Her favourite time was out-of-season Saturday lunchtimes when she would chat to locals as they ordered their favourite meals.

Many got to know that Jennifer was a nurse. Sometimes those lunchtimes felt and sounded more like a medical clinic... but in the nicest possible way.

She was occasionally tested by angry or impatient customers when things were running less than smoothly in the chippy. But she had the knack of quelling difficult situations.

One busy August evening, there was a little unrest among the waiting masses over the time it was taking to process orders because of a technical problem with the fryers.

A few customers walked away and sensing that things could get out of hand, Jennifer calmly called for hush and shouted:

'This is a small village fish and chip shop. We are doing our very best to serve you as fast as we can, and I can assure you it will be well worth the wait.'

No-one answered back, no-one else left the queue, in fact, virtually everyone praised Jennifer and the chip chop for 'doing a great job'.

Jennifer had the knack of getting us out of deep water with her remarkable 'keep going when all around you is falling apart' spirit.

Occasional crises from fryers not working to the chippy running out of cod, haddock and chips saw her put that rare and vastly underestimated quality to good use.

However, she was sorely tested on one unforgettable evening by a sudden flood that almost brought the chippy to a standstill.

We were in the middle of the school summer holidays and had just processed a hundred meals for a school group camping near Charmouth.

The queue to the takeaway was so long you could not see its end, and orders were coming in thick and fast when it became clear that water was pouring on to the chippy floor.

Aware that something was very wrong and getting worse, Jennifer kept her cool, continuing to serve customers with a smile.

Our friend and employee Ingrid was trying to process burger, pie and mushy pea orders at the rear of the chippy while standing in two inches of water.

The water was gushing from a tap that couldn't be turned off from an overflowing blocked sink. I frantically tried to stop the flow without success while continuing to cook.

Ingrid eventually managed to unblock the sink some fifteen

minutes after the flooding began. Customers were unaware there was a problem, even when the water started to rise.

Jennifer's diplomatic skills were frequently put to the test in the chippy, but particularly on one quiet April afternoon.

The lunchtime rush was over, there was no-one queuing for food, and Jennifer was taking a well-earned break.

I started a casual conversation with Ingrid about how safe it was for someone with one eye to drive a car or any other vehicle.

I told her my dad had passed his driving test with one eye. Although he had never had an accident, I joked that he had probably caused many crashes on the road.

Ingrid and I each covered one eye to see how good our vision would be with the other, coming to the conclusion that it would not be safe to drive.

We continued the conversation and hand-over-one-eye experiment as Jennifer returned to take a cod and chips order from a woman standing at the serving hatch.

Jennifer was trying to talk above us, commenting on how nice the weather was and asking the customer what her plans were for the day.

Jennifer had sensed, quite correctly, that my seemingly innocent chat with Ingrid was probably inappropriate in a public place.

It was just as the woman was leaving that Jennifer and I discovered just how unsuitable the conversation and gestures really were.

She said she had enjoyed listening to and watching us. But she wanted us to know that she had just one eye and drove very well and safely on the roads!

A dream home in the Trossachs

The view was breathtaking. Snow-capped mountains soared above the mirror-like waters of Loch Katrine. The sky was a brilliant blue and almost cloud free. We were totally absorbed by the vista from the holiday cottage we had booked in the tiny Trossachs community of Stronachlachar.

We knew we were lucky to be there.

Snow ploughs had cut a trail through snow more than two feet deep on an eleven mile single track road to the community just the day before we arrived.

For the preceding two weeks Stronachlachar had been completely isolated, with holidaymakers and the handful of residents stranded with dwindling food supplies.

We were only staying there because of a last-minute hotel cancellation on what was to be a twelve-day break in remote areas of Scotland.

I found and booked the Old Smiddy Cottage on the edge of Loch Katrine as a result of a quick-fire online alternative accommodation search.

Our four-day stay at this idyllic spot had a 'meant to be' feel to it, for it had a key role in shaping the rest of our lives.

We loved the peace and quiet, the beautiful scenery, being next to a loch steeped in history... and away from traffic jams.

Stronachlachar was – and still is – one of those rare places where you could walk for miles without seeing anyone else and not pass a car or vehicle of any kind.

It has a rich history steeped in the legend of Rob Roy MacGregor, born just a few miles from the community and immortalised in a Walter Scott novel.

We talked endlessly about selling our takeaway and cafe business in Dorset and moving to the Trossachs to escape the rat race.

In a personal journal, Jennifer wrote about the excitement of finding Stronachlachar and spending time there with me, her parents and her brother.

> *Paul has found us a real haven in Scotland – an old blacksmith's shop converted into a wonderful holiday cottage.*
>
> *The most amazing part is the loch, situated in front of us and surrounded by thousands of trees and snow-capped mountains... feeding our souls and spirits on an hourly basis.*
>
> *We have had four wonderful days here, watching the scenery change before our eyes. We have walked through areas bathed in sunshine and enjoyed a day of snow.*
>
> *This loch, this cottage, will stay in our hearts forever. We will take with us its peace and energy. And, God willing, Paul and I will find a way to return to this, our spiritual homeland, for good.*

On the final morning at the cottage, I wrote in the visitors' book that we had loved it so much we wanted to return – to live in Stronachlachar.

Just a few months later, Jennifer contacted the cottage owners, asking if there were any properties for sale in the area.

They replied almost instantly saying they were developing two new cottages. They planned to keep one as a holiday property and to sell the other. 'Would you be interested in buying it?' they asked.

Within a week we visited the area, toured the then shell of a home to be sold, put in an offer for it and had it accepted.

Just over a year after we first came to Stronachlachar we realised our dream, moving to a cottage developed on the site of an old laundry for the former Stronachlachar Hotel.

The purchase almost fell through at the eleventh hour when the sale of our business and home in Charmouth appeared to be in jeopardy.

Last-minute financial complications, emerging just a few days after we had sold virtually all the furniture and possessions in our house, put everything at risk.

We were sleeping on a blow up bed. Two deckchairs were our only seating in the lounge and boxes of personal items were scattered everywhere.

Crunch time arrived in March 2007. It was the afternoon and we were anxiously awaiting a phone call from our solicitor.

We knew that call would decide whether the financial issues had been settled and if the sale of our business and home was to proceed or not.

Jennifer and I were sitting on the deckchairs. We both fell asleep, tired from a busy morning at work and from having had the business on the market for almost two years.

We were suddenly woken by the phone ringing... and it was good news. The sale was going ahead and we could plan our new future in Scotland.

We moved to Stronachlachar on May 11, 2007, a day celebrated by Jennifer in writing in our personal journal.

> *I want to tell you about an amazing chapter in our journey through life. We have moved into our wonderful cottage on Loch Katrine.*
>
> *I can't believe that we are actually going to live here. Our garden is the Trossachs, the mountains, the rhododendrons, the local lochs and wildlife.*
>
> *It seems almost our destiny to have arrived here, particularly after our chance stay here last year. I hope this is the start of many good times. Scotland – I think we are home.*

We arrived with the help of Jennifer's brother, Stephen, and with the prospect of a few weeks' work locally at a newly opened tea room.

I continued to work there for eighteen months while Jennifer, continuously inspired by our move, built a new care consultancy business from scratch.

Her office overlooked our garden, in the early days a rough piece of ground riddled with rhododendron roots and topped with stones and poor soil.

Over a period of three years, Jennifer and I spent many hundreds of hours transforming it into a unique rock garden.

When we moved to Scotland, we ended up 500 miles away from our families in Devon and Somerset.

Some thought they would never see us again. Most started to visit us more often than when we lived a few miles apart in the South West of England.

It became a great holiday destination for Jennifer's parents and other relatives, and gave us important quality time together.

Jennifer and I were not the only ones who moved to Scotland. Willow, Jennifer's pet cat, was an important if initially reluctant newcomer to Stronachlachar.

She had been with Jennifer for fourteen years when she travelled up north. She was so upset about it all she didn't go out for the first year!

But, thanks to one or two hot summers, Willow gradually began to love spending time in our garden, particularly when we were outside.

When she died in 2011, we buried her in her favourite place – among the shrubs next to one of our favourite sitting areas.

Natural haven shaped from 'worthless' piece of ground

It was a shapeless piece of ground, riddled with rhododendron roots, thousands of weeds, broken parts of old brick, stone, old metal piping, yards of disused cable and rotting branches and pine needles from the dozens of trees surrounding our home.

Bordered by a driveway, fencing and decking leading up to our front door, this awkward, sorry-looking piece of land, untouched by human hand and uncultivated for decades, was our 'garden'. At first glance, it looked very much like a lost cause.

Transforming it was not a priority when we moved into our new cottage. In truth, we had no idea what to do with it or what could be done.

A few weeks after we moved in, Jennifer's brother, Stephen, did some 'messing about' in the garden, moving some old bits of wood and logs and walking up and down the site to get a feel for it. He found a lot of rocks, some loose, some firmly embedded in the ground.

With a small trowel he dug away at a corner of the garden, pulling away chunks of turf and a mass of moss and dandelions. Gradually, he started to unearth some beautifully contoured rock, stepped in such a way that it appeared to be part of a natural rockery.

Jennifer and I dubbed this little piece of exposed ground as 'Stephen's Hill'. We were amazed at the find, the smoothness of the rock, and the way a series of natural stepping stones had been uncovered, perhaps for the first time since the old Stronachlachar Hotel closed suddenly in 1939, or earlier.

During our first summer and autumn at Willow Cottage – named after Jennifer's tortoiseshell cat – we started to dig away at bits of ground nearest our home, finding more and more solid stone.

We were just curious about what was underneath all the earth and junk on the surface. Bit by bit, Jennifer and I revealed an amazing array of rock, working away at the ground with two small trowels, sturdy hand brushes and buckets to take away the detritus.

By the spring of 2008, we had 'explored' and cleared a third of the garden. We unearthed an incredible rockery with a natural pond, stone pathway and a series of nooks and crannies crying out to be planted in some way. Our discovery was beyond anything we could have imagined.

We still had no plan for the garden. Jennifer, who like me, had no experience in gardening of any kind, started sketching planting areas and visiting garden centres to see what would look nice and what could grow in our new little haven in the Trossachs.

She had a great vision – to create a tranquil outside space using traditional Scottish shrubs and plants in the main, and craft flowerbeds and areas of interest with slate and stone abandoned in a derelict old bowling green fifty yards away from our home.

Jennifer and I bought four large half whisky barrels and filled them with heathers and Alpine plants to give the garden definition and a splash of colour. We made flower boxes from old planks dumped nearby and used old roof slates and stone to construct interesting borders.

In the summer and autumn of 2008, we unearthed the middle part of the garden, shifting tons of earth and rubbish to expose more of the rockery and stone pathway. We rolled boulders into place to establish a large flowerbed and created one from the old slates.

This became our main outside seating area. Jennifer would spend hours here looking out over Loch Katrine. She was staggered by what we were achieving on a piece of land which was giving up its riches after being derelict for generations.

The following year, 2009, we tackled the third and final section of the land, moving two tons of stone to build a feature wall and putting in place the beginnings of a tiny wild garden, with a 'secret' sitting area which could not be seen from the cottage.

Jennifer turned the garden into a kaleidoscope of colour, growing many of our plants from seed in a tiny plastic greenhouse next to our home – from magnificent aquilegias of a variety of colours to sweet william, lobelia and poppies.

She was so proud when her first red poppy flowered magnificently in the spring of 2010. The joy of seeing it bloom is captured in one of my favourite pictures of Jennifer (see photograph section).

The garden matured with Zen-like qualities. It developed an oriental feel even though the majority of the plants in it are native to Scotland. Perhaps this happened because of the gentle curves and dips in the rockery, and the way Jennifer had planted it out.

In three years we shifted more than fifty tons of earth and debris to create our garden. We extracted miles of rhododendron 'tentacles' zig-zagged across every inch of the ground and removed enough pine needles and builders' waste to fill two skips.

Jennifer would always tell visitors and holidaymakers who fell in love with the garden that I had done the bulk of the work on it, particularly much of the landscaping. In reality, she did as much, if not more than me and was primarily responsible for making it so beautiful.

She developed green fingers she never knew she had. She spent many hours potting up young plants and transferring them to the garden. She had a clear view of how she wanted it to look and feel, introducing a sensory element to heighten the enjoyment of being in the garden.

She encouraged me to create vegetable boxes from old wood abandoned in nearby woodland. Within two years, Jennifer was growing everything from tomatoes, rocket salad and radishes to courgettes, celery, carrots, beetroot, onions, peas, broad beans and potatoes.

When we worked in the garden in the summer, many visitors probably thought we were aliens – or had something wrong with us. Midges, a real menace in the Trossachs between June and September, force you to wear protective clothing when toiling outside.

We would wear midge-proof head and body gear, attracting many strange glances from holidaymakers staying in holiday cottages. It was only when they had their less then gentle introduction to the mighty midge that they asked where they could get similar protective clothing!

Just a few months before she passed away, Jennifer re-organised the garden to make the most of the colour, height and texture of plants and shrubs. The garden was at its most glorious in her final summer, attracting large numbers of butterflies, finches and other small birds – and praise from tourists.

Jennifer was convinced the garden, with its waterside position and wealth of bird life, had 'healing' qualities. When she needed time to think, and respite from the many aches and pains she suffered, she would sit in the garden, even if it was raining or cold.

She found inspiration there for new work ideas, new challenges. The peace and tranquillity of this little piece of paradise were a great comfort to her, particularly in the last year of her life. Our garden will always be testament to her tenacity and love of nature.

2.

Courage in the face of great adversity

Perhaps once in a lifetime we encounter someone who has the ability to inspire us in one brief meeting, who can confront not one but two life-threatening illnesses with remarkable courage, and instil hope in others in the face of the greatest adversity.

Jennifer had all of those qualities, and so many more. She lived with a kidney transplant for twenty nine years and lung cancer for more than a year. She never gave in to illness, never lost her zest for life. Jennifer was without doubt the most courageous, determined, loving and kindest woman I have ever known.

Tributes that poured into our home in the Trossachs after she passed away suddenly in November 2013 described her as the *bravest, kindest, most loving, most inspirational* person they had ever met. Some of those accolades came from people who met her only once.

Jennifer had the rare ability to touch so many lives almost in an instant, to encourage people to live life to the full and to tackle pain, fear and danger with a smile. She inspired optimism in everyone she met.

She never gave up hope and never stopped helping others. Illness failed to break her indomitable spirit. She was a larger than life character who genuinely made every moment of her life count.

She constantly defied the odds to achieve great things, making her mark in home care throughout the UK and helping to transform the way we care for people with dementia, one of the greatest health challenges facing our society today.

Above all things, Jennifer was a loving daughter and sister and the most amazing wife any man could have. She put her heart and soul into a remarkable marriage truly made in heaven – and one that resulted in the happiest years of both our lives.

Jennifer suffered kidney failure as a teenager, enduring dialysis until, in 1984, at the age of twenty one, she had a kidney transplant at Southmead Hospital in Bristol. It marked a new lease of life for her, although she was told that the kidney may offer her only five to ten years of life.

Knowing that she may be lucky to reach the age of thirty, she graduated as a nurse two years after her transplant operation, fulfilling her childhood dream to follow in the footsteps of her grandmother.

She went on to become a senior hospital nurse, a care home and domiciliary care manager, a leading home care business adviser and trainer, and one of the UK's foremost experts on dementia care for elderly people living in their own homes.

Jennifer was determined that kidney disease, a transplant and medical care would not change or dominate her life. She adopted the same approach with immense success when she was diagnosed with lung cancer.

Only close family and friends knew about her illness. Jennifer made it absolutely clear that she wanted to be judged on merit not by her cancer. And extraordinarily, she reached new heights in her outstanding career in what proved to be the last year of her life.

Just a few weeks before cancer claimed her life, she gave key note addresses at two major conferences in the north of England, speaking so brilliantly and passionately about dementia care, and gaining ovations from appreciative audiences.

I saw her soar as a home care and dementia consultant, carrying out some of her finest work when she was 'dancing' with lung cancer and living with a deteriorating kidney, regular bouts of gout and swollen limbs.

She has a striking legacy, playing a pivotal role in raising awareness of and shaping better dementia care across the UK, and transforming the greatly renowned Dementia Gateway, the most important internet based dementia information service in the UK.

However great her attainments in her career, Jennifer and I would always tell you that our greatest achievement in life was to find and marry each other. Our love and devotion was, and will remain, unbreakable.

Her love of life was remarkable. She had an amazing, never ebbing strength that defied belief, driving her on even when she was exhausted physically and mentally. She always put on a brave face when she was ill, and was so good at it no-one would have guessed she was unwell.

Jennifer had qualities that are in all of us, but so few

demonstrate on a day-to-day basis. She was a constant reminder to me and so many others that humanity is important, being kind is important, caring is important, giving people time is important, listening is important.

I always said to Jennifer that I counted my blessings that we had met and married. Jennifer said that 'God had put me in her way'. She had no doubt that our relationship was written in the stars, was meant to be. That fate had intervened to bring us together.

Considering the incredible sequence of events that led to our first meeting, I would be the last person to argue with this. I know how lucky I was to share the best years of my life with her, but Jennifer would tell you that luck had nothing to do with it.

If I was asked to sum up my beautiful wife and the woman who inspired so many in a single sentence, I would use the ten short words from a thank you card from a hospital patient who had been looked after by Jennifer while she worked at Weston General Hospital in Weston-super-Mare.

They say real angels don't exist. But I've met one.

How right she was.

A dream shattered

We were just five days away from starting a genuine holiday of a lifetime to celebrate Jennifer's fiftieth birthday – a six-week break to see the wonders of New Zealand.

The flights were booked, the bags were packed and the excitement of beginning a tour of the North and South Islands that had taken almost a year to plan was building.

Jennifer, who had just celebrated the twenty-eighth anniversary of her kidney transplant, woke from a good night's sleep with a sharp pain in her chest, one that worried her enough to phone her renal consultant and arrange to see him.

It was unusual for Jennifer to be concerned about what she called a 'minor irritation', but she wanted to make sure she was fit and well for a potentially gruelling twenty-eight-hour flight to Auckland, the longest journey she had ever embarked on.

When we arrived at the hospital, Jennifer joked with the girls at the renal reception that there may be a ticket available for New Zealand if an examination she was about to undergo showed that she could not make the trip.

The consultant told her the pain was probably no more than a pulled muscle, but suggested she have a routine X-ray to give her peace of mind. The X-ray showed an abnormal mass in the lung, and a CT scan was arranged within the next hour.

The worry was etched on Jennifer's face, and no doubt on

mine. We just held each other as I assured her everything would be all right. We were both full of trepidation as the consultant called us in to discuss the result of the scan.

Seven earth-shattering words turned our world upside down. 'I am sorry, it's not good news,' he said. 'We can't be sure at this stage what it is, but we must get it checked out quickly,' the consultant told us. I only had to look at Jennifer to know she feared the worst – that she had lung cancer.

The shock was overwhelming. But amid the despair, she smiled and joked: 'Bang goes my chance of getting my pension then.' I was shaking as the consultant arranged for Jennifer to see a cancer specialist the next day.

We broke down uncontrollably in the waiting area of the renal unit of the Forth Valley Royal Hospital in Larbert, Stirlingshire. We hugged each other and wept there for more than an hour, totally inconsolable and unable to take in the enormity of it all.

Jennifer, always so strong, happy and positive in dealing with everything life had thrown at her, cried so deeply and asked in despair: 'What have I done to deserve this... why now, just as we are going to New Zealand?'

No words could comfort us. We couldn't face going home straight away, particularly as clothes and personal items purchased for a holiday that now seemed an impossible dream were scattered across virtually every room in our cottage.

We decided to get something to eat in a restaurant in Stirling. A waitress met us with a smile and asked so nicely and innocently what kind of day we were having. We didn't have the heart to tell her. 'It's been okay,' I said, fighting back the tears.

The diagnosis of lung cancer was confirmed just twenty-four hours later. The specialist said Jennifer's condition was 'serious but not hopeless'. There appeared to be two small tumours in the lung, and traces in the liver and spleen.

An operation was out of the question because of the position of one particular tumour – near the bronchus. He told Jennifer 'we are talking palliative care here'. So it was terminal. We didn't ask how long Jennifer might have to live.

Amid the raw emotion, we both knew our lives had changed forever in an instant. It was now clear that our trip to the other side of the world would have to be called off. A biopsy and other tests couldn't wait that long.

It was on our long drive home that we realised we would have to break the news to close family and friends almost immediately, and before we had the opportunity to come to terms with the impact of it all.

We had no choice because Jennifer's mum and dad were going to phone her on her fiftieth birthday which we were due to celebrate in a spectacular log cabin on the very edge of Milford Sound in Fiordland on New Zealand's South Island.

We were going to call my sister who was undergoing an operation to remove cancerous cells from her womb as we were due to fly from Heathrow to Singapore on the first part of our journey to the other side of the world.

My son David, living in Auckland after emigrating there in 2011, and so looking forward to seeing us for the first time in more than two years, was due to collect us from the airport on our arrival in the city.

Telling them our devastating news was the hardest thing we ever had to do. We then had to get away, booking a cottage near Loch Lomond to escape the madness of it all, and to think about what was in store for us now.

The biopsy showed that Jennifer had a rare, slow-growing non-small cell cancer that affects younger women who have never smoked. Encouragingly, she was told there was a chance she could be offered a revolutionary new genetic treatment.

Jennifer was tested for suitability for taking *Tarceva Erlotinib*, an oral drug only just licensed for use in Scotland and already proven to be effective in shrinking tumours and enabling people to live well with lung cancer.

Only 7% of people with Jennifer's type of cancer have the right genetic make-up to benefit from the drug. We hoped so strongly that she would be in that minority, particularly as the alternative, chemotherapy, could damage her kidney.

Fortunately Jennifer was among the 7%. Treatment started almost immediately and kept Jennifer well for more than a year. There were many days and weeks when her health was so good I almost forgot that she had lung cancer.

The timing of the diagnosis could not have been worse. But it was a blessing in disguise. The cancer may not have been detected for several months if the routine check-up for a chest pain – which had nothing to do with the cancer – had not happened.

Jennifer, showing no symptoms at the time, may well have been diagnosed when the cancer had been at a much more advanced stage, seriously reducing her quality of life and perhaps shortening her time on this earth.

If we had gone to New Zealand, the long and arduous flight there could in itself have caused complications. This is all speculation but Jennifer and I agreed that an early diagnosis was almost certainly the lesser of the evils.

We didn't get to Milford Sound, but celebrated Jennifer's birthday in style in a cliff-top cottage overlooking the sea and spectacular Assynt Mountains in the tiny hamlet of Nedd, near Drumbeg in North West Scotland.

A remarkable anniversary

Jennifer could not have been happier. We had booked a room for a very special anniversary at our favourite hotel. As we dressed for a celebration dinner, we cracked open a bottle of champagne and raised our glasses to 'Fred', Jennifer's transplanted kidney.

We were marking a remarkable milestone, the twenty-ninth anniversary of Jennifer's kidney transplant operation. Through her great courage and positive attitude, she had defied all the odds to reach this point in her life, including living with lung cancer for almost a year.

This moment of great celebration at the Rufflets Hotel, near St Andrews, was also a poignant one for Jennifer. She knew she would not have been alive but for receiving the kidney from a young man who had died tragically in a road accident in the South West of England.

So, as we toasted Jennifer's triumph, we also lit a candle and said a prayer for the young man's family to remember the loss and sorrow they had endured, and to thank him for the gift of life he had made in death to Jennifer.

Jennifer had been on dialysis for more than two years –

with the help of a machine at her then home in Clevedon in Somerset for much of that time – when she received the 'perfect match' of a kidney in October 1984.

A trainee nurse at Bristol's Frenchay Hospital, she was rushed to the nearby Southmead Hospital for the four-hour operation. Just twenty-one at the time, she was full of hope – but also fearful – about what her future would now hold.

The day after the operation, she received a letter from the chaplain at Frenchay, Father Bob Torrens, who told her: *When news of your transplant came through, there were whoops of delight. It was very clear to me that they love and appreciate you a lot.*

Jennifer was told that a kidney from a deceased donor typically lasted between five and twelve years. So to reach a landmark twenty-nine years, making her one of the longest surviving kidney transplant patients in the UK, was no ordinary achievement.

Jennifer's incredible determination and will to succeed helped her to survive and thrive in those years. She never gave up hope, smiled through periods of poor health and took on challenges that many believed were beyond her.

Her sense of humour helped her through many difficult times. She often joked about her health, made light of cramps and pains and frequently had fun with me and others when talking about her transplant.

Just a few days after our first date, she said she needed to tell me about a long standing bond with Fred. She told me they had been together for more than seventeen years and she couldn't live without him.

She looked me in the eye and asked: 'Do you have a problem with that? Fred will always be with me. He's a vital part of my life. He keeps me going, looks after me...and I would die without him'.

My face must have been a picture. I was imagining that Jennifer was asking me to have a relationship with her while she was engaged in a long standing romance with a bloke called Fred.

She laughed out loud as I told her I did not want to be involved in a *ménage a trois*, explaining that Fred was not someone she was seeing but was the name she had given to her kidney!

I used to watch and marvel at the positive impact she had people on dialysis and those who had recently undergone transplant operations when I accompanied her on regular visits to hospital kidney units at Southmead, and in Glasgow and Stirlingshire.

She loved helping others including Kate, a teenager from Bristol who had just had a kidney transplant, having been on dialysis for three years. Kate was worried about the medical regime she would now be on, the potential side effects, and the longevity of her kidney.

At that stage Jennifer had had her transplant for more than twenty years, and been a patient at Southmead since her operation. She was having an iron infusion when she chatted to Kate about how long she had had her kidney, and all the things she had done in her life.

Kate's spirit lifted almost immediately. She was so enthused and astonished at meeting someone who had had a transplant for so long. She said it was the best tonic she had ever had – a line often repeated by the many who met and spoke with Jennifer.

Jennifer revelled in telling her story, knowing that it could only inspire and help others on dialysis and awaiting a transplant, and those who had recently received a donor kidney. She had the ability to transform people's lives in just a few short moments.

Jennifer had the nickname 'happiness whirlwind', and for good reason. She livened up normally sedate renal clinics where people were waiting anxiously for appointments, perhaps chatting quietly with partners or friends, and constantly looking at watches to check the time.

She would burst into the waiting area full of life and laughter, joking with reception staff and nurses carrying out blood tests. She would always make them smile while telling them about the highlights in her life, about her work, and about me.

She kept the same happy spirit when she met the consultant, taking good and bad news on the chin, always listening, but always determined to take everything in her stride and not let her health issues get in the way of enjoying life.

Jennifer adopted that same indomitable spirit in her move to Scotland, encouraging people on dialysis and new transplant patients. She always found time to talk to them, to tell them about her experiences, and never failed to make them smile and be more positive.

The happiness whirlwind weaved the same magic in the oncology unit at Forth Valley Royal Hospital, walking into the unit with a big smile, cracking jokes with reception staff and nurses, and speaking so eloquently and forthrightly with specialists.

The oncology unit is the one place people are happy to walk past as they arrive for appointments at the hospital. I was so impressed at how Jennifer would turn that walk into a positive, almost everyday experience.

Before our last holiday together, Jennifer, in her own special way, told renal and cancer consultants that we were going on a break to North West Scotland, and she was sure nothing would get in the way of that! It was her polite way of saying that she would be going come what may.

Her transplant anniversary was celebrated in a different way every year we were together, with a special cake, champagne, a meal for two at a nice restaurant, a short break in a holiday cottage or a get-together with friends and family.

The seventeenth anniversary included a memorable interview on Radio Bristol when Jennifer announced that we were due to get engaged twenty-five days later, and she hadn't made up her mind whether to accept my proposal of marriage!

What she didn't tell me or anyone else was that she would ask me to marry her at our engagement party held in Burnham-on-Sea the night before her thirty-ninth birthday. That was Jennifer – always full of wonderful surprises.

She was so well in those days, not even daunted by taking on the fish and chip takeaway in Dorset. She enjoyed putting in long hours and never took one day off sick at the takeaway, even during or after the grinding peak summer period.

When she had a slight cough and lost her voice one July, she refused to take time off or see a doctor or her renal consultant at Southmead Hospital. When she was eventually persuaded to have it checked out, she was told she had had pneumonia. The doctor was amazed that she had worked through the illness.

There were more local radio interviews on the twentieth and twenty-fifth anniversaries of her transplant. On the twenty-first anniversary, Jennifer wrote about her transplant in a private journal in which we shared important memories and milestones in our lives.

It's an unbelievable achievement, she commented. I was told when I had the operation that five years was regarded as a success and ten years as a miracle. So now, I wonder what would be said about twenty-one years.

My thoughts are very much with my donor and his family. Twenty-one years of life also means twenty-one years that they have not been able to share. The parallel between life and death is sometimes a strange one.

The biggest and most significant change in my life is my husband, Paul. He has completed my dream of finding true love, mutual respect and happiness. His presence in my life can only enhance the life of my kidney.

So who knows what happens next. Ten years was said to be a miracle. With all this happiness and love nurturing me and my kidney, perhaps I could reach thirty years with it. Who would have believed that?

On the twenty-ninth anniversary of her transplant, Jennifer did what she always did. She told as many people as she could to inspire them, enthusiastically announcing via online kidney support groups that she would soon be joining an exclusive 'thirty club'.

Today I want to send a huge thank you to all the dedicated doctors and nurses at Southmead who helped me during the first twenty-two years, and then to Glasgow and Forth Valley Royal Hospitals in Scotland who have looked after me in the remaining years, she wrote.

I send out my thoughts to the person who chose to give me a chance by signing their kidney donor card and to his family for supporting that decision. Celebrate with me by telling someone close how much you care and do something special just for yourself. Life is precious, don't waste it.

Her messages – spread across numerous renal transplant sites – produced dozens of positive responses from people who were amazed that Jennifer had achieved three times the longevity she was told to expect.

Jennifer did more than she could ever know to further the cause of transplants, encouraging people to become donors, and inspiring so many on dialysis and after having a transplant. Her longevity, positivity and fighting spirit was the greatest encouragement to everyone who met her.

Her kidney did not fail once in those twenty-nine years. Jennifer excelled in defying expert opinion, believing that the power of the mind and spirit could overcome any obstacle put in her way.

Who could argue with that?

The brave 'dance' with cancer

It's a diagnosis no-one wants. You hear the words 'you have incurable, inoperable lung cancer', but they don't really sink in straight away. The words seem so final, so devastating, and so cruel.

In the space of a few seconds, your whole life is turned upside down. The future you planned and hoped for is snatched away. Hopes of growing old together are gone forever.

The tears flowed. Jennifer and I shook with emotion and fear. We looked at each other in silence for a few moments, hugged so tightly and whispered 'I love you' to each other almost simultaneously.

'I'm sorry, I won't be growing old with you,' Jennifer told me. 'I am going to cause you so much pain, so much heartache.' I was distressed that she would have to endure another major crisis after facing so many other health challenges.

In the hours and days ahead, we talked about the future and how best we could spend our precious time together. Jennifer was absolutely clear about one thing – terminal cancer was not going to get in the way of us enjoying life to the full.

Getting the go-ahead to take the breakthrough genetic drug

treatment, *Tarceva Erlotinib*, proved the key to enabling her to fulfil all the things she wanted to do – and more.

The decision to tell only close family and friends that she was 'dancing with cancer' – her very own way of describing how she was living with the illness – proved critical to her wellbeing and professional life.

She knew people who had been treated with kid gloves or 'overlooked amid a well of sympathy' when they had told employers or business clients they had cancer or another serious illness.

Professionally, Jennifer wanted to be judged on merit not by a disease. She was involved in ground-breaking dementia work and did not want the focus taken away from that.

It was tough for her – and for me – seeing this through, particularly on days when she was coughing up blood, feeling low or suffering from gout and swollen limbs.

Two months before she passed away, Jennifer wrote about her cancer in the personal journal we had kept since we became engaged twelve years earlier.

I knew nothing about the entry until I found the journal in the drawer of her office desk three weeks after she passed away. I still can't read the words without breaking down.

Here is what Jennifer wrote:

September 4, 2013

It seems amazing to me that this is the next entry in our diary given the year we have endured. But this book has always been written in when the time was right. So I console myself with that thought. For some reason today is the day I can write about our epic year.

Read this entry slowly as it will take you through every emotion. It starts in October 2012. We had been planning for over six months the holiday of a lifetime. We were going to New Zealand to celebrate my fiftieth birthday.

We were staying for six weeks and would travel the North and South islands. Paul had found amazing accommodation and we had planned all the places we would visit and all the things we wanted to experience...

Milford Sound in a log cabin for my birthday, the Bay of Islands, Fiordland, Rotorua, Dunedin and many others...

The weekend before I was due to go, I had a sharp pain in my chest, left and side. Of course, as a nurse, I immediately thought heart attack!

I was due to visit the kidney clinic to check bloods, meds etc before we made the journey. Everything seemed fine but my doctor suggested we do a chest X-ray and ECG just to double check.

Tests were routine. I didn't feel unwell and we talked more and more about New Zealand. The long flight scared me a little, but I was looking forward to stopping in Singapore and visiting the botanical gardens to see all their lovely orchids and the excitement of landing in Auckland and seeing Paul's son David and his partner, Laura.

At fifty years old I was going to the other side of the world. I couldn't quite believe it or that I would have six glorious weeks with Paul. I looked at my husband and counted my blessings. All my dreams had come true.

We went back to see the renal consultant to get the results. The kidney clinic was quiet. It was the afternoon and I joked with the girls on renal reception that if I was not well enough to go there could well be a ticket going begging!

Somewhere deep inside me I knew we were waiting too long. If the news had been good my consultant would have come bouncing out. When he did come out I saw his face – a man who was preparing himself to shatter another person's world.

He asked Paul and I to come in. Thankfully he came to the point. I remember the words – I am sorry it's not good news. At that point your heart beats a little faster. Your brain stalls like a train and the rooms seems to be in a bubble where everything is still.

Next – we have found a mass in your chest. We can't be sure at this stage what it is but we must get it checked out quickly.

I responded like most people – with disbelief, and tried to attribute it to a previous bout of pneumonia. It must be scarring. Perhaps it's hereditary.

But I knew this was not good. Most likely I had cancer. I looked at Paul, tears in his eyes, trying to be strong, but inside his heart, like mine, was breaking up into a thousand pieces.

I said I am so sorry. Sorry for not being able to go to New Zealand. Sorry for not having our dream holiday. Sorry you will not see your son. But mostly sorry because I was going to cause him so much pain now and in the future.

Like others, I had a million and one questions. How could this be happening? I am so well. We are soulmates. I have gained so much love in my life. I don't want it to end. I am not ready to leave.

In the reception, I broke down uncontrollably. Paul held me tight, stayed strong. The girls there rushed round to support us. The consultant looked and I know felt our pain and I am sure must have struggled, knowing he was the one who had changed our world.

When we later drove home, Paul tried to convince us it was okay; a benign tumour, scarring, something hereditary. He looked at me and said: 'You think it's cancer, don't you?' I couldn't lie. In my heart I knew, but I couldn't take hope away from anyone.

The next day back to the hospital to see the lung specialist, Dr Peter Wright. In my sleep the night before, I felt a gentle presence. I had a vision that I had lung cancer and it was inoperable. But I was being assured it would be okay.

I was then the frail human sitting in front of the specialist. After a look at the scan, he said: 'You have lung cancer. It has spread to your liver and spleen. It is serious, but not hopeless.'

He matter of factly went through the options – chemotherapy, radiotherapy, palliative care. We cried and held each other's hands tightly. Once again, I said sorry to Paul. We spent an hour and a half with Macmillan lung cancer specialist Jennifer Wilson, discussing everything, looking for reassurance and listening.

She told us about the possibility of a targeted therapy – Tarceva Erlotinib – an oral tablet that you take once a day. You can stay at home. It has good results. I needed to be EGFR positive and have a certain type of cancer (non-small cell lung cancer). The chances were slim. Less than 7%.

I discovered that some non-small cell lung cancers have particular mutations which lead to uncontrolled cell growth and the formation of tumours. They include EGFR, or epidermal growth factor receptors. Erlotinib works by blocking EGFR in the cancer cells. Don't ask me why but I felt it was going to be okay. I will be in that 7%.

Next was the biopsy. I chose to have it in the liver because I feared they might collapse my lung. Paul, as Paul does, got to work to make sure my birthday would be good. He found an amazing house perched on a cliff edge – Sea Horses in Drumbeg, Sutherland, and booked it for a week.

Telling the family...

Paul and I always take whatever life throws at us, deal with it and then present it to the family with all the information to answer their questions. This time it was different. Everyone knew we were going to New Zealand. David and Laura were meeting us.

Paul's sister, who had been diagnosed with womb cancer, was having her op – we were ringing her family from Singapore.

We picked up the phone and gently told all of them. We took our time. Leading them slowly up to the moment when we would change their world in the same way ours had been. But in a quicker, more brutal way.

Jennifer was very much a *Tarceva* pioneer. She was believed to be the first long-term kidney transplant patient in Scotland to be taking the drug, so her reaction to it was of considerable interest to cancer specialists and research scientists.

Jennifer was prescribed the drug just over a month after being diagnosed with lung cancer. She took it once a day in the morning and was advised of possible side effects, specifically a rash, nausea, tiredness and diahorrhea.

She developed a rash within a few days of starting the treatment. It spread across her chest, face and into her scalp.

But she was told that this was probably a good thing, a sign that *Tarceva* was beginning to work.

She kept a daily treatment diary, recording the appearance and spread of the rash, days when she felt excessively tired and nauseous, and how it led to changes in medication she was taking daily to regulate her kidney. The rash disappeared after a few weeks.

She had regular CT scans at Forth Valley Royal Hospital to check how she was responding to the treatment. Between Christmas 2012 and the summer of 2013 there were clear signs that she was doing well.

Early scans showed that the tumours in her lung had shrunk and that there appeared to be no traces of cancer in her liver and spleen. The results were a huge boost for both of us and for family and friends.

The scans were carried out without the use of a dye (contrast medium) injected into the bloodstream because of the risk of it affecting Jennifer's kidney function. Contrast medium would have given more accurate results, but it was clear that she was reacting well to *Tarceva*.

In August 2013 we took a well earned break in an idyllic cottage at Tarbetness, near Portmahomack in North East Scotland. It was a haven of peace and quiet in the height of summer, with seals, herons and gulls being our only company.

On the long drive home, Jennifer coughed up a small amount of blood. It was the first time this had happened and it worried her. We drove straight to the casualty unit at Forth Valley Royal Hospital for a check-up.

When we returned home, a fresh CT scan was arranged. It showed that the tumours in Jennifer's lung had grown, but by small amounts. She was advised *Tarceva's* effectiveness in combating the cancer may have been reduced.

Her consultant talked to her about the possibility of taking another drug, *Afatinib*, a biological therapy for non-small cell lung cancer – or a Mark II *Tarceva*, if you like – that was still in the trials process at that stage.

The consultant later confirmed that funding had been secured to allow Jennifer to take *Afatinib*, perhaps later in 2013. She would be one of very few in the UK to be prescribed the drug. Again, this gave us great encouragement.

She joined online lung cancer support groups, to find out more about the *Tarceva* treatment and to offer support and encouragement to other people living with cancer and a kidney transplant.

The following extract from a conversation she had with the daughter of a woman 'battling' with lung cancer after having a transplant, offers an insight into how she coped with life threatening illness.

I always say I am living or dancing with lung cancer rather than dying from it. I do not talk in terms of battles or struggles as I feel these are very negative thoughts and suggests that one of you will lose.

I prefer to think of my cancer as a rose that has shed a few petals in my body. The petals have been picked up with the rose remaining and...as long as we regularly prune it back it will stay in check and we will rub along together, which suits me fine.

I sometimes think that it is harder for loved ones rather than for the person who has the condition. They imagine how we feel, what we have to face, and whether we are in pain, and are putting on a brave face.

One of my kidney doctors gave me excellent advice. He said you are likely to have many worries (particularly

because I am also a nurse) in relation to your kidney,
treatment and life. For each worry he suggested that I ask
myself: Can I do anything about it today? If so, do it. If
not, put it in a box until you or your medical team can
help you.

Over all my years with my transplant, I have had
many doctors trying to work out the secret of its longevity.
To be honest, it comes down to one thing; positive thinking.
Truly believing that your kidney will survive and you will
have a long life. I have adopted exactly the same policy
with cancer.

Jennifer never allowed the cancer or conditions linked to her
kidney disease to stop her from carrying out her important
work.

She often did talks, presentations and workshops when she
was unwell. She attended meetings and conferences when she
was struggling with pain.

Jennifer frequently worked on her laptop and took business
calls from her bed when she should really have been resting.

I, of course, expressed my concern about all of this. But I
knew it was what Jennifer wanted to do, and no-one, including
me, was going to tell her she could not do something.

Her incredible spirit, doggedness and stubbornness had
helped her achieve such longevity after her kidney transplant.
She was not going to allow cancer to dictate how she lived and
worked.

We always worked side by side and attended meetings and
all events together. We were as one in everything we did. While
I supported her on our travels and in meetings, conferences and
workshops, I was in awe of her energy and brilliance.

Wherever we went, I was the only one who knew of the

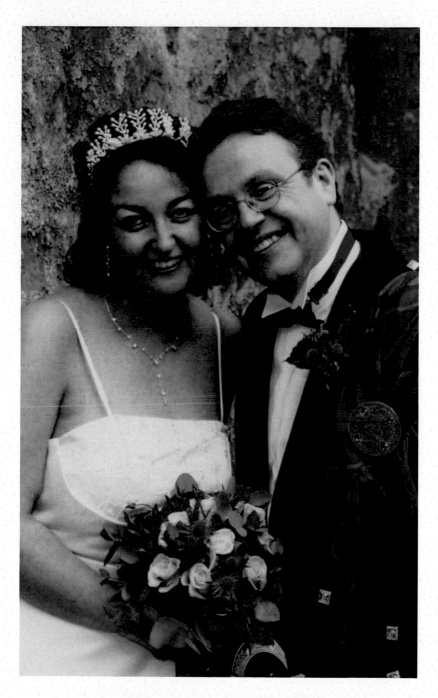

Our dream wedding at Dundas Castle, near Edinburgh in 2003.
Picture by Norma Ann Photography, Glasgow.

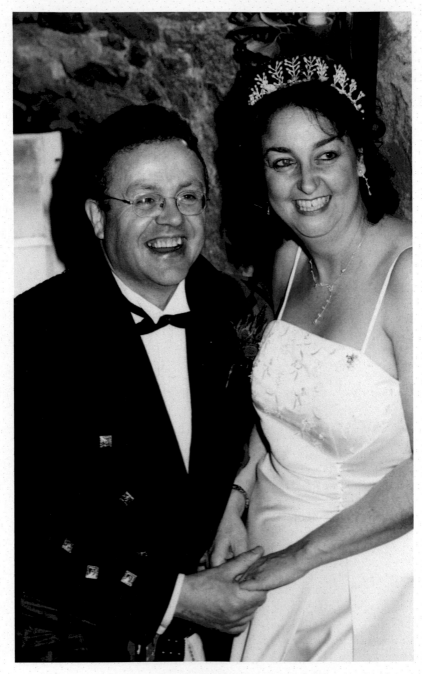

So happy…on the steps leading up the Auld Keep at Dundas Castle. Picture by Norma Ann Photography, Glasgow.

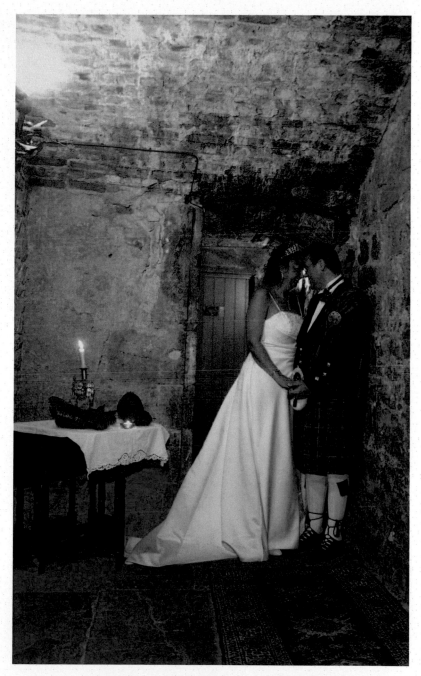

So close...in the Auld Keep at Dundas Castle.
Picture by Norma Ann Photography, Glasgow.

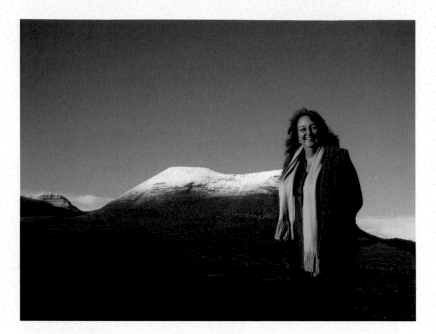

Jennifer in the Highlands just after her 50th birthday.

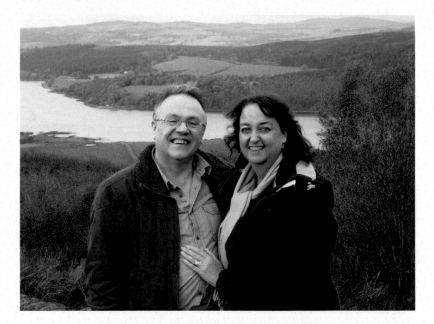

*Paul and Jennifer heading for Drumbeg in the Highlands
to celebrate Jennifer's 50th birthday.*

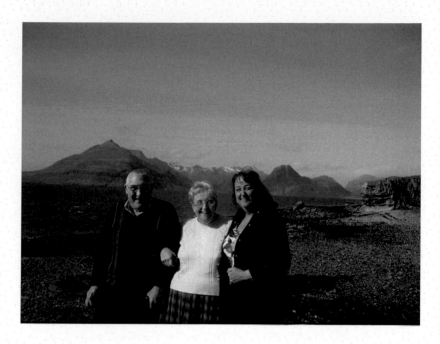

Jennifer and her parents, Glyn and Joan Dark, in Elgol, Skye.

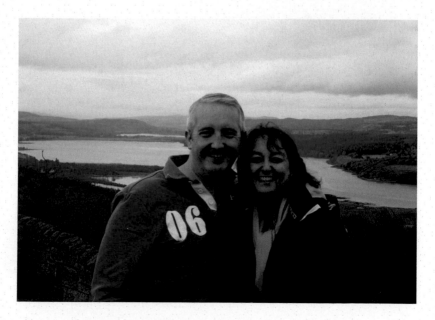

Jennifer and her brother Stephen in the Highlands.

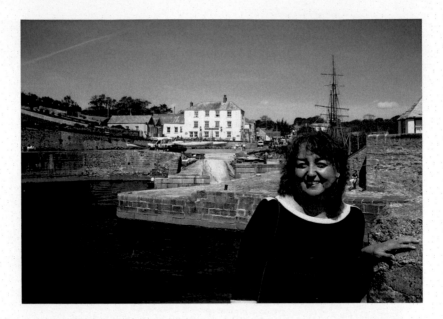

Jennifer in picturesque Charlestown in Cornwall in May 2013.

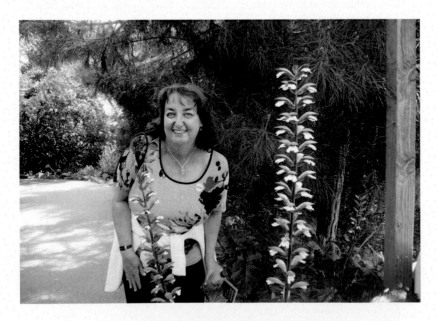

Enjoying a visit to the Eden Project in Cornwall in May 2013.

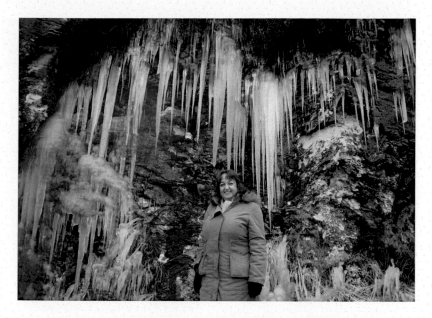

Jennifer under a cathedral of icicles in Stronachlachar in 2010.

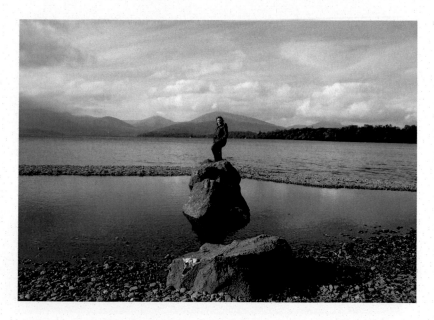

The sun shines on Jennifer at beautiful Balmaha on Loch Lomond — just days after being told she had lung cancer.

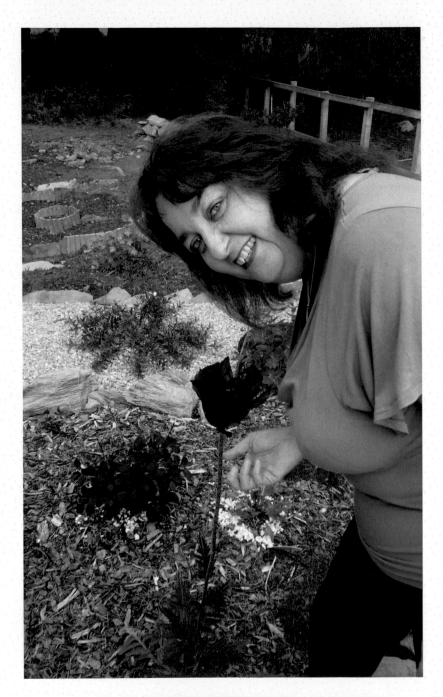

So proud of her first poppy in our garden in Stronachlachar.

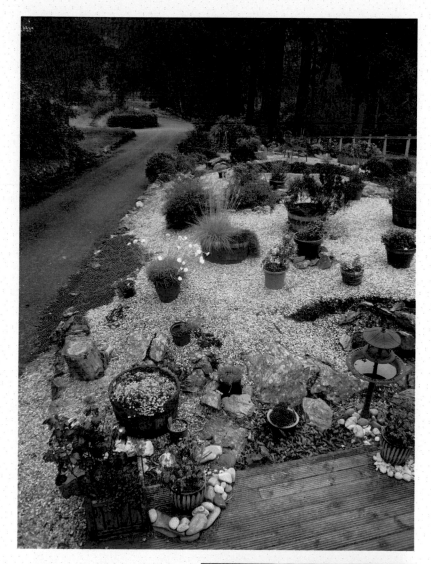

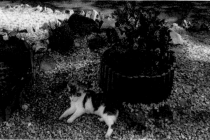

*Above: Our garden in 2014
– created with much love
and devotion.*

*Right: Willow basking in the
sunshine.*

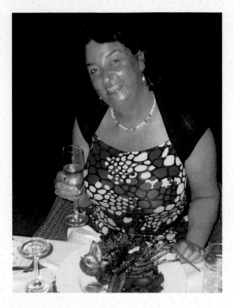

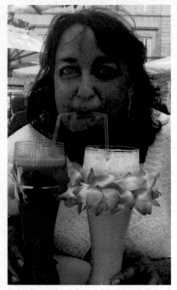

A lobster dinner to celebrate our 5th wedding anniversary in the Maldives.

Having fun and a drink or two in Carcassone.

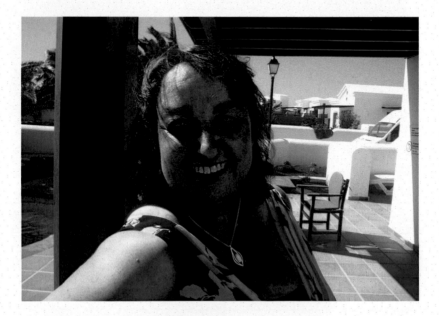

Celebrating our 10th wedding anniversary – Jennifer in Lanzarote.

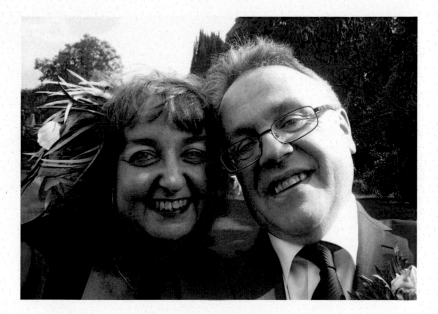

So much in love...attending a family wedding in Devon in 2011.

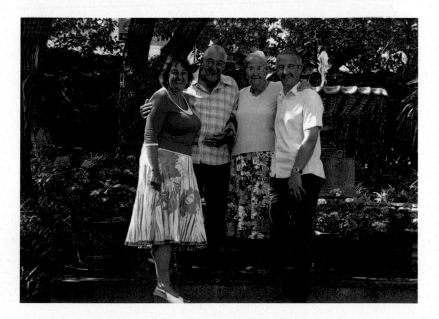

*Jennifer with her brother and parents as they celebrated
their Golden Wedding in Madeira in 2008.*

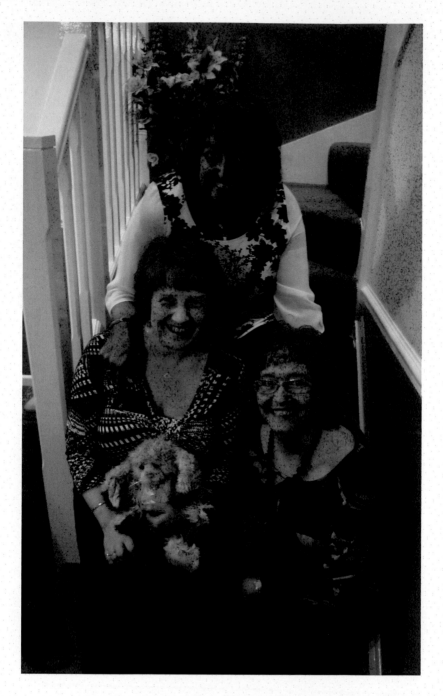

Jennifer with her cousins Sally and Mary in 2013.

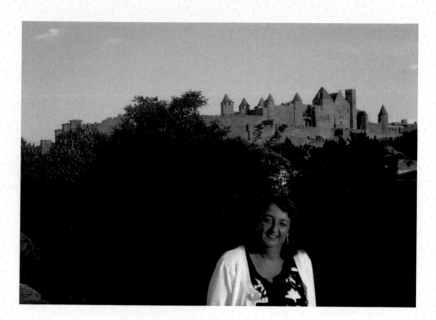

Jennifer outside the walled city of Carcassone.

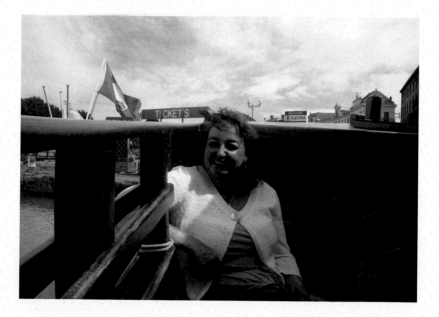

Relaxing on a boat on the Canal du Midi near Narbonne in France.

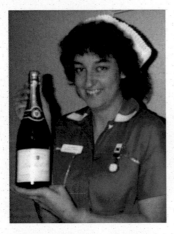

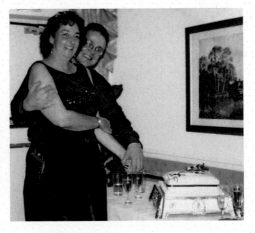

Celebrating with champagne...
Jennifer graduating as a nurse.

Cutting the cake to mark our engagement
in 2001.

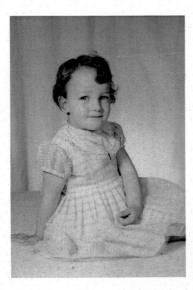

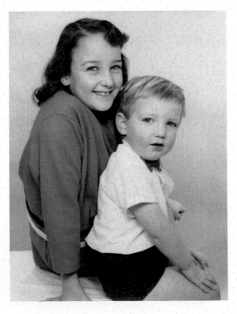

Jennifer as a toddler. Picture by
Eric Purchase, Wells.

Jennifer and Stephen. Picture by
Eric Purchase, Wells.

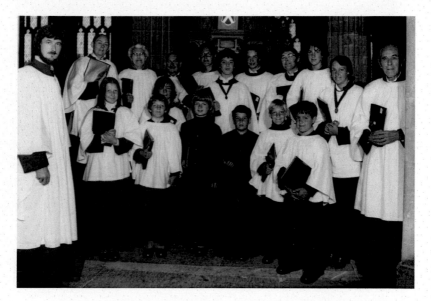

St Cuthbert's Church Choir, Wells, with Jennifer in the back row (second right).

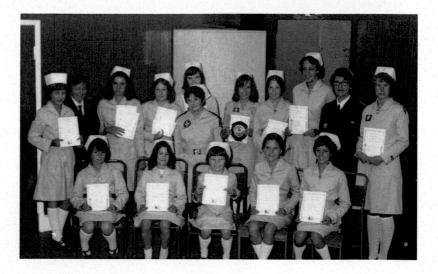

St John Ambulance cadets in Wells, with Jennifer (back row, third right) and her cousin Sally (back row, fourth right).

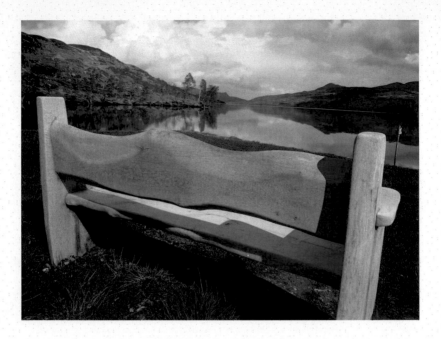

Jennifer's bench at Stronachlachar, overlooking Loch Katrine.

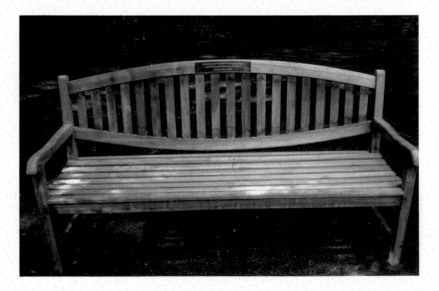

*The memorial bench at the Bishop's Palace gardens
in Wells, Somerset.*

enormous health challenges she was facing, and the effort she made to look and sound well. It was so hard at times to contain my emotions as Jennifer addressed audiences, knowing what she was enduring.

She took poor health in her stride, never shirking any challenges, never crying off from attending events she had promised to speak at.

As much as she loved her work and doing it well, Jennifer's greatest joy was spending quality time with me at home and on holidays.

In our last year together, we took two breaks in the Canary Islands and explored many of the more remote coastal areas of Scotland.

The first holiday abroad, in Playa Blanca, Lanzarote, was to celebrate our tenth wedding anniversary. We renewed our marriage vows. Jennifer planned and filmed the whole event.

Our last holiday was in Torridon in North West Scotland where we immersed ourselves in each other, staying in a beautiful lochside house, and at Melfort Village, near Oban.

Jennifer's medical notes made it crystal clear she had terminal cancer. But she never gave up hope of living well with it and for a number of years. We fervently believed that, together, we could overcome any crisis and achieve anything we wanted to in life.

Even when she suffered a collapsed lung on the third day of our last holiday together near Oban, she was absolutely convinced she would pull through. A scan showing the cancer had spread to her liver and that she had pneumonia in her left lung was not enough to dent her spirit or will to live.

She was a patient at the Forth Valley Royal Hospital when plans were made to shrink a growing tumour in her bronchus through radiotherapy.

We spoke about her returning home after her treatment, almost certainly with the help of oxygen and probably with palliative care.

On Jennifer's fifth day in hospital, I sent an email to my son, David, who was living in New Zealand, to tell him what was happening.

I wrote:

Things have been particularly difficult here in Scotland in the past week. As you know, Jenny and I started a two-week holiday on October 26. We went to the North West Highlands for a week and had a fantastic time, even though the weather was blustery. Jenny has been a little short of energy recently, so we just read books, had long lie-ins and enjoyed the house.

On Saturday, November 2 we moved to a pretty little place called Melfort Village, near Oban. Jenny's brother, Steve, joined us there for the week. Jenny by then was much better. She dipped a little on Sunday, but was better again by Monday morning.

During the afternoon, she started to cough up small amounts of blood and this did not stop. Later that day, we took her to the A&E at Oban. After investigations, they admitted her and gave her oxygen to stop the coughing and calm her. The following day she was taken by road ambulance to the Forth Valley Royal Hospital – our local hospital.

From there on she underwent a series of tests, scans and other investigations to try to get to the bottom of problems affecting her. The scans established that Jenny had suffered a collapsed left lung. Things were complicated by poor liver and kidney function, so she became seriously ill.

The scan also showed that cancer had spread to her liver and that the tumours in her left lung had started to grow again. Essentially, the Tarceva treatment she has been on since last November had started to become less effective. After many more investigations by oncology, renal and respiratory specialists, it has now been agreed that Jenny receive targeted radiotherapy treatment for a tumour sitting near the bronchus and affecting Jenny's ability to breathe. At the same time she is being treated for an infection caused by a mucous block in her lung. Jenny's kidney and liver function remains poor.

She is drained after a taxing few days. Steve has been a rock getting me to and from hospital and helping me to cope with the unfolding events. Jenny is going to Glasgow on Sunday to get her one-off radiotherapy treatment on Monday and will be returning to Forth Valley Hospital later that day. It is hoped that this will help improve Jenny's breathing and clear up the infection.

Funding is in place for Jenny to move on to the next stage of Tarceva treatment which is still in its trial stages. The success of the radiotherapy and in dealing with the infection is key to Jenny being able to take Tarceva Mk 2 (Afatinib). Jenny is hoping to be able to return home once they have got to grips with the infection. She will need oxygen and other support and is now very keen to come home.

It's been a traumatic few days. Jenny's resolve and massive will power to stay well and live with cancer has been sorely tested, and it's been an emotional rollercoaster for her, me, Steve and Jenny's parents. In the past year we have lived with the knowledge that something like this could happen, but nothing prepares you for it.

As you can imagine, there is a lot riding on the next few days. We both know that our time together may well be very limited – we have known that for the past year. Jenny is putting quality of life above everything else. She doesn't want to be continuously attached to monitors and a multitude of tubes.

What has been agreed for the next few days is Jenny's plan. She has been absolutely amazing. Her courage in the face of extreme difficulty is humbling. Jenny is determined to do all she can to achieve quality in life and remains positive about the future. We don't know how long we have got together now – none of us do in reality. But we want to make the most of every moment we share.

Jennifer passed away suddenly less than twenty-four hours after I sent the email, and two days before she was due to have radiotherapy. I was with her at the time. The shock was overwhelming.

I could not believe that my beautiful, courageous wife had had her 'last dance' with cancer. It felt as if I had died that day too.

But the brutal truth is that Jennifer had the kindest exit she could have hoped for. If she had survived, she almost certainly would have needed constant medical care.

Her kidney was starting to fail, the cancer was rampant and her body was struggling to cope with the demands being put on it.

Two days before she passed away, Jennifer had told me and her brother, Stephen, that she didn't want to be in hospital and wired to monitoring machines for any length of time.

She got her wish, but in such a devastating way.

Kindness personified

It was a cold winter's morning and snow-capped mountains and frost-covered fields provided a picturesque backdrop for our journey to Glasgow. We were on the way to a city hotel to deliver a six-hour dementia workshop for home care workers and managers.

Travelling by train from Stirling, we were just settling into our seats when Jennifer noticed an elderly woman passenger in apparent distress. Sitting on her own, she was frantically searching her pockets and through her handbag and started to cry.

Jennifer walked over to the woman, sat next to her and asked if she could help. The woman said she was looking for her daughter but hadn't been able to find her. She didn't have any money for her ticket and was worried she would be 'kicked off' the train.

Jennifer discovered in a conversation with the seventy-two-year-old woman that she had early stage dementia, and had got on the train mistakenly at Stirling while waiting for the arrival of her daughter, her son-in-law and three grandchildren from Newcastle-upon-Tyne.

Jennifer calmed her down, assuring her everything would be all right and paid for her fare to the next available stop at Falkirk, where we all got off the train and headed back to Stirling, staying with her at the station until her daughter and family arrived.

It was a happy ending to a potential crisis for a vulnerable woman. Jennifer stepped in to provide help when it was really needed. The family were so grateful that she had, and we still arrived in Glasgow in plenty of time for the workshop.

That was the measure of my remarkable wife.

She always thought of other people first even when cancer was taking its toll. In the last few months of her life, she spent many hours helping relatives of an aunty living with pancreatic cancer, talking to them on the phone or offering advice and comfort in private Facebook conversations.

She supported another aunty looking after an aged husband with Alzheimer's disease, seeing her when she could and offering practical help and advice to put her mind at ease, particularly before and after visits to a GP and admissions to hospital.

Jennifer was a tower of strength to a neighbour in Stronachlachar living with terminal cancer, visiting her at least once a week, keeping in touch with her via Facebook and helping her in her home. Like Jennifer, the neighbour was a trained nurse and greatly welcomed her support.

Jennifer supported me when my eldest sister died from undiagnosed colon cancer in November 2012, just a few weeks after Jennifer was diagnosed with lung cancer. She helped me draft a tribute to my sister and encouraged me to read it to a large congregation at her funeral.

When I was diagnosed with Type 2 diabetes, Jennifer inspired me to completely change my diet to keep it under control. This was no mean feat. I was known as the 'pudding monster' because of my 'ability' to eat huge quantities of sugar-rich food in a day.

I would consume a large packet of chocolate biscuits while watching a rugby match. My idea of a treat was a four litre tub of ice cream with two to three apple pies thrown in. It was not unusual for me to eat four to six items from a restaurant dessert menu, one after the other.

When Jennifer and I married, she arranged for me to be served with a gigantic ice cream and fruit dish – the size of a large punch bowl – as a joke at our wedding breakfast, thinking I would give up after a few spoonfuls. To her surprise I ate the whole lot and still found room for some of her mother's cranachan!

Jennifer helped me to switch to a sugar-free diet, to take more exercise and accompanied me on all my visits to my diabetic nurse. Without her support, I am not sure I would have had the will power to change my eating habits so quickly and so effectively.

Just a few months before she died, I faced the prospect of losing all my teeth after being diagnosed with severe periodontal disease, exacerbated by my diabetes. Jennifer emboldened me to seek the right treatment and came with me for my first appointment.

For me, it was not a priority, particularly as Jennifer was living with lung cancer. I was prepared to face a future with dentures, but she would have none of it. I was so moved by her determination for me to 'get it sorted', I continued the treatment after she passed away.

Jennifer was a constant inspiration to me, helping me to achieve great things with her – at work and at home. She introduced me to the world of home care and dementia, valuing and making the most of my experience as a writer as she established a consultancy business.

She helped me to value everything I did and that of others, and to be a better person. She showed me what it is like to be truly loved and to enjoy a 'slow life', celebrating all the good things that made us tick.

Jennifer regularly organised surprise holidays for both of us including one to the Maldives to celebrate my fiftieth birthday. Just two months before she died, she arranged for her brother to go on a challenging 4x4 driving course in rural Scotland, something he had always wanted to do.

Jennifer organised a family holiday in Lanzarote in her final year to ensure her parents celebrated their fifty-fifth wedding anniversary in style. She also arranged for her dad to try out a disability scooter on the island, knowing that he was about to give up driving. It gave him a new lease of life.

Jennifer touched so many lives without even knowing it. She motivated friends, family and countless others to make the most of their lives, to be happy and grateful for good health. Her infectious smile and magnetic personality were a welcome tonic for anyone meeting her.

She was never miserable or complained about the cards she had been dealt in life. For her, they were a reason to defy the odds. There were days when she was too tired or unwell to get out of bed, but I could count them on one hand in the years we had together.

A genuine
Good Samaritan

The sun was shining over Loch Katrine as the last customers at the waterside tea room said their goodbyes. It was almost 5pm on a quiet, uneventful Saturday in August 2007.

It was our first summer in Stronachlachar – and what a good one it was – and Jennifer and I were running the newly opened tea room at the local pier for a couple who were having a day off.

The tables were cleared, all the dishes had been washed, the floor had been mopped and cleaned and we were about to close for the day when a woman in a hurry burst through the doors to tell us: 'Please don't shut... there's been an accident.'

It transpired that a coach with fifty people on board had gone off the narrow B829 half a mile away, wrecking the vehicle's front axle. No-one had been injured but the coach was blocking the highway to all other vehicles, including a second single-decker bus with another fifty passengers.

We reported the incident to the police, but with us being in such a remote rural area it quickly became clear that no-one would be racing to the rescue in a hurry, or that repairs would be carried out to the damaged vehicle anytime that day or evening.

So, within the next hour, we had one hundred people from the two coaches descending on the tea room. They were worried, frustrated, thirsty, hungry and had no idea when they would be able to leave. We were asked to provide meals and drinks for them all.

We were not sure we could cater for them all as supplies were low. The tea room was in those days very small, able to sit up to thirty people, and there were just three of us working there that day – Jennifer, me and a teenage neighbour who helped out at weekends.

Jennifer was not daunted by the scale of the challenge ahead. After checking what food we had left and what we could provide she recruited six volunteers from the coach passengers with catering experience, putting them to work in the kitchen to help prepare food and wash dishes.

Within two hours, Jennifer worked a near miracle in feeding everyone in three sittings, making the most of the supplies available, and doing it all with a smile and happy background music. She chatted to as many people as she could telling everyone what was being done.

She received a rousing round of applause from very grateful stranded passengers at the end of the evening as they were ferried to the nearest village, Aberfoyle, by replacement minibuses that had been able to negotiate an alternative unclassified route around Loch Katrine.

I was staggered that we had been able to cook and provide drinks for so many people at such short notice and with seemingly few provisions in fridges and freezers. I was equally astounded at how a small band of volunteers had been able to gel as a team so well and so quickly.

It worked so well because everyone warmed to Jennifer, her coolness and ability to get things done. Jennifer explained that she was like a swan – calm and serene above water and paddling like mad underneath to stay afloat! She never panicked or believed that catering for so many was beyond us.

When other people hesitated in stepping in to aid someone, or just walked away, Jennifer would not hesitate to offer assistance. If someone was looking lost or lonely she would take time to ask if they were okay, and if there was anything she could do to help them.

During a weekend visit to her parents' home in Wells, Somerset, Jennifer and I went to the local cinema to see *The Golden Compass*. As we left the auditorium, she noticed a sad-looking woman walking slowly and alone just a few yards behind us.

She engaged her in conversation, finding out that she had been to see the same film but didn't like going to the cinema on her own. She was amazed that a complete stranger – Jennifer – had taken the time to talk to her. She said it was the first time anyone had shown interest in her in months.

Jennifer had that rare gift so few people demonstrate these days – kindness. It oozed through every pore of her. Jennifer, who had an ancestor called Kindness, was passionate about life, about living every moment and every day as if it were her last.

Ill health from a young age had taught her not to waste any moment of her precious life, not to be negative in any way. She was very much a glass half full person. If there were ten negatives about doing something and one positive, Jennifer would hang on to that one positive.

She made people feel good, special. When she talked to someone she made them feel they were the most important person on earth. She encouraged everyone she met, helping them to strive for something better, to always believe that this was possible.

She had immense charisma. People liked her, what she had to say and how she said it, always with a message of hope. Jennifer always found time to help someone, to do a good deed. She never asked or looked for thanks or reward. She just loved helping others in any way she could and was so trusting.

A great communicator, she put vulnerable people at ease – a great asset in her career as a nurse and care executive. Nothing was too much trouble for her, from assisting people with shopping to going to the aid of motorists in broken down cars. Of course, it made her vulnerable at times. But Jennifer remained undaunted, preferring to look for the good in all situations.

An elderly woman walking around Morrisons supermarket in Stirling and struggling to identify and collect food for her shopping basket will never forget her. The woman was using a magnifying glass to spot items she needed, and had a stoop that prevented her from reaching up to shelves.

Jennifer spotted her, offered to do her shopping and spent the next hour patiently walking around the supermarket with her. She then helped the woman through the till and Jennifer and I loaded her shopping into a taxi to take her home.

When we ran the takeaway in Dorset, we had great admiration for the courage and determination shown by an elderly man with Parkinson's disease.

Every Saturday lunchtime, Fred would walk the 300 yards from his home to the takeaway to order fish and chips, sometimes taking an hour to get there and back.

When he was no longer able to make the journey, Jennifer would take the food round to his home, taking time to sit with him while he ate and have a conversation.

He was forever grateful to Jennifer, calling her his own guardian angel for finding those valuable moments to look after him.

She was dubbed an 'angel' when she came to the rescue of an elderly man struggling for change at a parking meter in Stirling. He needed £2.50 for a ticket and had only 50p in his pocket. He looked around at the impatient queue behind him and whispered 'Sorry.'

Jennifer gave him the £2 to get his ticket and then helped him to his car with his three bags of shopping.

He asked for her address so he could send the money to her. Jennifer told him: 'That's on me – I might need you to help me one day.' He was so grateful he hugged her and planted a kiss on her cheek. Again, he could not believe that a stranger would come to his aid.

Jennifer was born in Wells and District Hospital in Somerset just after midnight on October 28, 1962.

The daughter of Glyn and Joan Dark, she attended Wells Junior and Blue Schools before going to Strode College in Street to gain the examinations she would need to be a trainee nurse.

She was a happy and precocious child, always looking to help in her family's bakery shop in St Cuthbert Street, Wells.

She once got herself in hot water when she pretended to be her mum in ordering supplies for the shop by phone. She asked for more than the usual number of doughnuts, and her punishment was to eat the extra ones in one go!

She liked talking over the fence to neighbours as a young girl giving a running commentary on things happening in her family household.

She enjoyed looking after her younger brother Stephen, and took charge of her younger cousins Sally and Mary when they went to the local park.

Jennifer loved singing and joined the choir at St Cuthbert's Church in Wells, becoming head chorister as a teenager. She went on to become a member of an eight-piece Motown tribute band – Band of Gold – which had a popular following in the Bristol area in the 1980s.

She loved walking, particularly in and around Stronachlachar, and reading books and magazines was a great passion of hers.

She loved cats particularly Willow who she rescued from an animal sanctuary near Bristol. Willow was with her for eighteen years, longer than any partner she had had, including me. They were inseparable.

She enjoyed going to the cinema and theatre and was fascinated by the characterisations and real-life situations played out in the TV soaps *Coronation Street* and *Emmerdale* and in political dramas.

Eating out was a great joy for Jennifer. She had a penchant for virtually every variety of seafood, and loved dining at the Loch Fyne Oyster Bar on the road to Inveraray and at remote seafood restaurants in the Highlands.

A career inspired by St John Ambulance

Jennifer's courage and determination to make a success of her life was evident in her teenage years when she became a trainee nurse just a few months after being diagnosed with kidney disease.

From a very young age, she wanted to follow in the footsteps of her grandmother, Martha Annie May House, who had been a mental health nurse in Somerset before the Second World War.

Illness, dialysis and a kidney transplant, and concerns among family and friends over her health, were not going to stop Jennifer from fulfilling that ambition.

Jennifer had shown her aptitude for caring as a young member of St John Ambulance in Wells, practicing on family members, particularly her brother and dad.

They 'volunteered' for bandaging and 'first aid' support as she passed examinations in a wide range of subjects, including 'casualty simulation' and 'preliminary home nursing'.

She became a trainee nurse in 1981 at Frenchay Hospital, Bristol, impressing doctors, senior nurses and her colleagues with her immense enthusiasm, positive attitude and her love of caring for other people.

Jennifer never wanted to let anyone down, often battling with and frequently overcoming exhaustion and poor health to demonstrate that she could and would be a good nurse.

She was so tired after one night shift she mistakenly posted a shopping list to her mother, taking the letter intended for her to Tesco's where she discovered her error.

Patients loved her smile, her kindness and ability to get things done. She worked hard and built a good relationship with – and won the respect of – fellow nurses and doctors.

Her qualification as a Registered General Nurse was not just a personal triumph, it was a day of great celebration for her family, friends and fellow nurses who had shared her journey to this new pinnacle in her career.

Anne Hitchens, who trained with Jennifer as a nurse, said she was a 'mother hen' to young nurses, 'fussing over us and giving us guidance on not drinking too much and maybe getting some sleep once in a while'!

Anne said Jennifer coped with sickness from kidney disease so well that 'most people didn't know she was sick at all, until she had had her transplant.

'Nowadays she may not have been allowed to have continued, but as she was so keen to be a nurse, and so good at it, the night sisters would make up beds for her in the linen cupboards (as she struggled with exhaustion) to ensure she got her "time in" on night shift. They would not have done this for anyone who was not deserving of it.

'Jennifer was also great at motivating people to go that extra inch. One Christmas Eve she persuaded a bunch of us to dress up as Muppets to hand out gifts to the children on the wards. Jennifer was "Big Bird", I was "Animal". Jennifer just loved to make people happy.'

Her first position as a junior staff nurse was in Frenchay's orthopaedic ward. She was twenty-three and marking the second anniversary of her kidney transplant which had given her the energy needed to carry out a demanding role.

Within a few months she moved closer to home, to Weston-super-Mare's Weston General Hospital, working in the female surgical ward before being appointed senior staff nurse/acting sister in the same ward.

It was as a young nurse that Jennifer learned one of the most important lessons in her life – that there is always time to deal with a crisis and that time is the greatest gift you can give to anyone.

A bed alarm had gone off in her ward. A woman patient was suffering a heart attack and Jennifer had raced to her side to help, only beaten to the bed by the ward's 'tea lady'.

Jennifer remembered being 'all fingers and thumbs', semi-panicking about providing the right help while she awaited the arrival of a doctor who saw she was 'in a bit of a state'.

The woman's life was saved and Jennifer was called into the doctor's office. She said she had been worried about the lack of time she had to do anything in the three minutes she awaited his arrival.

The doctor asked her to stand still in his office for three minutes and do nothing. It dawned on Jennifer how long that time could feel – and how much could be done in those valuable minutes.

It helped her to become a better nurse, to be calm and to offer effective support at the right time. It also proved invaluable in helping her to deal with crises in her professional and personal life.

Jennifer, at the age of twenty-five, became a sister at the Fountains Nursing Home in Weston-super-Mare, a senior staff nurse at St Mary's Hospital in Clifton, near Bristol and then a sister at the city's Abbots Leigh Nursing Home.

At twenty-seven, she took a bold move into home care, then an unregulated industry. She became a senior manager for three major companies, helping them to grow their businesses and play a key role in giving home care greater kudos in the UK.

She first started working with the United Kingdom Home Care Association (UKHCA) in the 1990s when it was very much a fledgling association, established to give a national voice to the many disparate home care providers across, England, Wales, Scotland and Northern Ireland.

Jennifer developed and delivered business development and other workshops. She produced detailed home care and dementia training packages for UKHCA members, and was appointed the association's independent complaints adviser in 1997.

Lesley Rimmer, OBE, former chief executive of the UKHCA, said she first recruited Jennifer as a regional development officer after she initially served on the board while working as a regional manager for a large home care provider.

Jennifer offered the rare combination of first-hand knowledge of the delivery of domiciliary care with an understanding of the policy framework in which the services operated, and had the skills to help with the overall development of the sector and the organisation itself.

Lesley said:

'In all the years I worked with Jennifer, I never had occasion to regret her appointment to the staff. She helped with so many different things in so many different ways and personally supported me in difficult times. But, mostly, I remember her for the laughter.

'Only a couple of weeks before she passed away, she rang

me to tell me of the sudden death of Margaret Rhodes, the former UKHCA treasurer. As well as the inevitable sadness at Margaret's passing, we laughed all over again at some of the situations we had found ourselves in.

'We were recalling that while a board meeting was held in London before Christmas, several of us had decided to go to Harrods. We took a bus and Margaret and I took a double seat together. I was on the outside and the combination of two well-padded rears made going round corners a risky mission. We laughed all the way there.

'Jennifer was always very professional. Despite the fact that she was unwell, she got Paul (me) to bring her to mid Wales to do a workshop. Seeing how unwell she was, UKHCA general manager Peter Randall and I took turns to give her half hour breaks during the day to recover her voice while we 'winged it' on vaguely associated topics.

'I think it is true to say that the four of us knew that the event was very nearly cancelled at the last minute and my appreciation of her determination to do her job come what may was enormous. Equally importantly, it made me focus on the need to have a 'plan b' if at all possible, something which I was grateful for when a speaker couldn't get to a Northern Ireland conference because he had forgotten his passport and couldn't fly. You know who you are!

'I remember going to Glasgow with Jennifer to conduct interviews for the role of Scottish Development Officer. My personal secretary at the time booked the hotel for our accommodation and for the interviews. When I told the then UKHCA secretary which hotel we were booked into, he said "You can't stay there." But my secretary would not budge – she had seen the brochure and said it was fine. So off Jennifer and I flew – separately.

'Jennifer got there before me. She walked in to find the manager about to put his fingers into a live light socket. In her normal way, she said "I'm a nurse and I don't think you ought to do that." She persuaded him to leave it and then asked for some tea. While providing this, the manager told her that the chef had walked out a few days earlier so there were no meals available in the hotel, but there was a bar next door.

'It was around this point that I came in hot foot from the airport. It was something in the way Jennifer sat me down and said "I'll get you some tea," which made me realise all may not be well. Luckily, we laughed at the lack of food and unfurnished nature of the hotel and met the UKHCA secretary Dr John Womersley for dinner – out of the hotel.

'We waited for him in the bar next door which was rather rough and ready and the only place that I really have heard someone say "Hey you, Jimmy."

'John came in and said "We are not staying here." And marched us off.

'Breakfast time was a delight. There was no hot food except toast and even the suggestion that he might scramble some eggs sent the manager into meltdown. And then we went to see the interview room. And things went from bad to worse.

'It was in a basement with no natural light and smelt of damp. We were not having that. What an advert for an organisation to interview in such a venue. So we sat upstairs in the corner of the lounge and went to the deli to get sandwiches for lunch.

'The hotel waiter – who bore a striking resemblance to Manuel in *Fawlty Towers* – kept interrupting our attempts to interview, to be told by Jennifer: "Not now!" in strong tones.

'At the end of the day she and I walked back down through the centre of Glasgow in total hysterics at the happenings of the previous twenty-four hours. We never failed to remind each other of it. It was just so funny and, more to the point, we survived!

'What I will miss most is her reminding me of the good times we had and hearing her laughter.

'She always said I was not good at hiding what I thought. I have apparently a repertoire of "looks" which I dispense to those who displease or bore me.

'If she could see me now she would see a look of sadness on my face, tempered by the fact that I know she lived by the rubric '*carpe diem*', and did indeed live every day as if it were her last. She will be sorely missed.'

Jennifer ventured into new territory in 1998, helping to establish a business selling the concept of sound wave therapy for pain relief and stress reduction. The experience proved pivotal in encouraging her to launch further successful enterprises.

These included the internet based Caring for your Business, which specialised in helping home care providers to develop niche services, to embrace personalised care and to be at the vanguard of providing better care for people with dementia.

She also launched Roberts Consultants, an enterprise she started from scratch specifically to help new or struggling home care businesses to develop new services and to understand how marketing and good branding could help them thrive in a difficult environment.

Over the years, through 'troubleshooting' clinics, face-to-face meetings, workshops and seminars, countless numbers of businessmen and women have benefited from her experience and her absolute belief that care is the most important profession of all.

Her welcoming smile, kindness, great personality and ability to inspire others brought her considerable success and plaudits. More importantly, those rare and enduring qualities endeared her to all those who met her, even if the meeting was fleeting.

She was never arrogant, ruthless or dismissive of others. She worked hard and was a good listener and communicator. Her philosophy of treating everyone as she would want to be treated paid so many dividends. I never encountered anyone who had a bad word to say about her.

She thought on her feet and was rarely unable to offer the right advice at the right time. She always found time to answer a query or offer timely advice or a potential solution to a particular problem, even when she was at the point of exhaustion and feeling less than well.

The same characteristics that shaped her early years, and led to her becoming a nurse and highly respected home care and dementia professional, held her in good stead throughout her life. Anyone who met Jennifer just once or knew her well will never forget her.

Presenter and trainer par excellence

Jennifer had been unwell for a number of weeks. She was suffering from gout in her hands and wrists, her ankles were badly swollen because of poor circulation and she was struggling to eat and sleep.

A recent CT scan had revealed that the tumours in her left lung were growing. She had been advised that the medication she had been taking to combat the cancer was becoming 'less effective', and an alternative would have to be considered.

But nothing was going to stop Jennifer doing what she loved – spending quality time with me and carrying out dementia work that was so important to her wellbeing and to her ever flourishing career.

It was October 9, 2013, exactly a month before she passed away, that she talked so passionately, eloquently and brilliantly about dementia and vision at a regional care conference at the Cedar Court Hotel in Wakefield.

Jennifer spoke on her feet for forty-five minutes without notes. She engaged a diverse audience, making people laugh and keen to learn and listen. She was on top form and it was a joy to watch and experience.

The following day, Jennifer was a guest speaker at a similar conference at Blackpool's Hilton Hotel. Again, she put in a memorable performance, using humour and her vast experience to illustrate the importance of good vision for people with dementia.

She summoned up all her courage and determination to do those talks and no-one hearing her, apart from myself, would have been aware of her health problems. That was the mark of Jennifer. She never gave up or gave in to poor health.

In my long career as a journalist and care consultant, I have heard hundreds of speakers at public and private events, attended many lectures and seen countless presentations by government ministers, MPs, health experts and business leaders.

Jennifer was one of the best speakers I have ever heard. You may think I am biased, but I am basing this judgment on twelve years of working with and listening to her at national and regional conferences and other events across the UK.

Jennifer always had ovations after her talks and presentations. She always topped 'best speaker' polls conducted at the end of major conferences and workshops. And she always left stages and podiums with applause and words of praise ringing in her ears.

She had the rare ability to connect with individuals in an audience of any size, from a handful of people to an auditorium of hundreds. People listening to her for the first or umpteenth time liked her and enjoyed her performance.

She was inspirational in so many ways in what she had to say, how she said it and how she made people feel. She had the 'wow' factor and left a lasting, extremely positive impression on everyone she met.

Jennifer's approach echoed the words of African-American

poet, actress and civil rights activist Maya Angelou: 'People will forget what you said. People will forget what you did. But people will never forget how you made them feel'.

No-one was ever left in any doubt that she cared passionately about her expert subjects – home care and dementia.

Jennifer frequently talked without notes and with little aid from electronic presentations. She liked the personal touch, regularly referring to everyday situations in her life to illustrate or clarify a particular point.

Her experience as a nurse, as a long-term kidney transplant patient and a successful business woman and care consultant, proved invaluable in delivering key presentations on home and hospital care and dementia.

Jennifer wrote, produced and delivered dozens of training courses for the UKHCA focusing on home care, dementia awareness, business development, and troubleshooting and handling complaints.

They were always delivered with great aplomb and professionalism. There were a plethora of tributes to her work, and queues of delegates wanting to catch a word with her at the end of each event.

I have seen her turn unresponsive, cynical and downtrodden home care audiences into reinvigorated individuals ready to face the challenges of tomorrow because of what they had heard and learned from Jennifer.

I have watched with admiration as Jennifer took the 'hot seat' in problem solving clinics, answering and dealing with often complex questions covering a range of issues from the difficult behaviour of people with dementia, to ways of developing new and niche businesses.

What made her so different and so special? What helped her to stand out from the crowd? Why was there a clamour to talk to her after her presentations and lectures? What made her a genuine champion of home care and dementia?

She had the rare ability to engage with everyone from all walks of life from professors, doctors and nurses to care home owners, managers and home care workers. She talked in terms everyone could understand and encouraged everyone she met.

It helped her that she had overcome so many hurdles in her own life, particularly her kidney disease and transplant and associated health issues. Her near thirty years of experience in home care and dementia care also proved invaluable.

She genuinely knew her subject well. She had real-life experience of caring for people, particularly those with dementia. She spent many hundreds of hours talking to people with dementia and their carers to understand what they needed to live well with the condition.

Jennifer talked about her uncle and how he coped with Alzheimer's disease (although never naming him to protect his privacy). She learned from his experiences, his behaviour patterns and response to medication to advise on providing better care for people with dementia.

I had only known Jennifer for a few weeks when I had the opportunity to see her in action, to watch her enthral audiences with her humour and real-life experiences. And to witness at first hand her determination to not let illness get in her way.

She asked me to drive her to Wales to deliver a home care workshop. She had a dreadful cold, a temperature and felt nauseous throughout the day. With these symptoms, most people would have stayed in bed. But Jennifer, with the help of UKHCA executives, continued to deliver the six-hour workshop in her own inimitable way.

I supplied her with copious amounts of water to keep her going. She never lost her way, answered every question fired at her and had attendees queuing up to speak to her at the end of the session to praise her presentation and get advice on a number of issues.

I supported her at all events from then on, sometimes speaking alongside her on media issues, occasionally acting as her 'technical assistant' for electronic presentations and frequently dealing with administrative matters at conferences and workshops.

She always exceeded people's expectations, particularly in training sessions. She knew how to 'win over' sometimes reticent audiences. Most of all, she loved doing this work and her great knowledge and infectious enthusiasm were obvious to all.

Jennifer was innovative not just in her approach, but in producing and delivering unique training sessions on dementia and vision, dementia and dentistry and the thorny subject of how home care companies should handle complaints from clients.

She was in great demand. So much so that two leading organisations, the UKHCA and the leading eye care company, VisionCall, appointed her as their dementia lead with many more increasingly seeking her expertise.

Remarkably, many of her key appointments came after she was diagnosed with lung cancer. She soared in her career rather than letting illness get the better of her. She truly turned great adversity into triumph.

3.

Dementia visionary

John was terrified every time a plane flew over his village home in Devon. The frail pensioner crawled under a table or hid in the wooden shed at the bottom of his garden until he could no longer see or hear the aircraft.

Friends and neighbours often found him shaking and crying, with his hands covering his ears to try and block out the noise of the plane engines. They thought he was going mad and did not know how to help him.

John had no close family and refused to see a doctor or seek help. When John's health started to deteriorate, an old friend of his shared his concerns with villagers over a pint at his local pub on Exmoor.

I happened to be in the pub at the time and overheard John's sad tale. I left my contact details with his friend, advising him that 'I might know someone who can help'.

He looked me up and down and just said: 'Right.'

Two days later, completely out of the blue, he contacted me, initially criticising me for listening in to a private conversation. He then asked how I could help and I put him in touch with Jennifer who was fascinated by John's story.

Jennifer and I visited his friend, Brian, in Tiverton. We talked about John, his life, his home and his experiences. 'He won't see you or talk to you,' Brian insisted. 'He's an awkward sod at the best of times.'

When we got to John's home he was sitting in his garden. He shouted: 'I don't want to buy anything,' as Jennifer got out of her car and walked towards his home.

She told him: 'That's good... I'm not here to sell you anything.'

He was intrigued by this woman he hadn't met before. 'Have you come to take me away?' he asked.

'No,' said Jennifer. 'I'm doing some research about the village and I'm told you are the best man to talk to.' Not exactly the truth, but it broke the ice.

Jennifer and John sat on a garden bench, talking for more than an hour about the village and about his memories. He told how he grew up in London in the 1930s and 1940s before being evacuated to the South West of England as a twelve-year-old.

When Jennifer asked him about the bombing raids on the capital he became very agitated, asking her to leave. He calmed down when she changed the subject, but had difficulty following and remembering their conversation.

He had vivid memories of the distant past – as a boy, getting his first job delivering bread and moving to Devon in his youth – but he struggled to recount anything he had done that day or in the previous week.

Jennifer believed John had dementia. And that the planes

flying over his home were a horrible reminder of the bombing raids on London which he and his family had endured before he was evacuated to the country.

She discovered that John and his family took refuge in an old Anderson shelter at the bottom of their garden during the raids, thus explaining why he hid under a table or in the shed at his current home when planes flew over.

She talked this over with his friends and neighbours who were able to encourage him to see his GP. He was diagnosed with Alzheimer's disease. He was given home support – and the opportunity to escape his fear of planes.

Jennifer discovered that the aircraft scaring him were low flying RAF jets on training manoeuvres. The flights usually took place once a fortnight, on Wednesdays, when John was at home doing some gardening or watching TV.

Jennifer encouraged friends to take him out for the day on Wednesdays, to the shops in Barnstaple, to the seafront at Ilfracombe or Lynmouth or to local libraries where they would read through old papers or books about Exmoor.

Six months later, Brian contacted Jennifer to tell her that John was 'a new man'. He was having treatment for his Alzheimer's disease, loved his days out and no longer hid under his table or in his garden shed.

John's story is a microcosm of Jennifer's approach to dementia. She believed, quite rightly, that people can live well with dementia and that there are rational explanations for – and solutions to – difficult or unusual behaviour.

A care home contacted her about a resident who was causing havoc twice a day, seven days a week. At 7am and 4pm, he was 'climbing the walls' of his room and a communal lounge, shouting that he had to get outside.

The resident, a man in his 70s, had dementia. His problem

behaviour had baffled staff and the care home manager and was upsetting others living there. He became isolated and his health suffered as he shunned meals and drinks.

Jennifer watched him for a day. She talked to him and his family about his life and found out he had been a milkman on a farm for more than twenty years, a job he enjoyed and was sorry to have to give up when he retired. He had been used to bringing in cows from the fields for milking at 7am and 4pm.

With Jennifer's help, the home arranged for him to visit a local farm twice daily as cows were brought in for milking. It gave him a new lease of life, ended his difficult behaviour in the care home and brought him back into contact with other residents.

During a dementia workshop she was delivering for home care workers, Jennifer was told about an elderly man with dementia who was living on his own and would only allow one care worker into his home to look after him.

Jennifer spoke to the care worker, noticing she wore a distinctive red hair band. She said the elderly man she cared for had told her several times he liked the hair band, adding that it was similar to one worn by his late wife.

Other care workers, previously not even allowed through the door of the man's home, were able to provide support for him when they took Jennifer's advice and started to wear the same hair band – or showed it through his letter box on their arrival.

At another workshop, Jennifer was told about a kind and gentle elderly woman who started swearing at home care staff and her family. They were shocked and bewildered by her behaviour for none of them had ever heard her use foul language.

Jennifer spent several hours with her and her family. She

believed the woman had undiagnosed frontotemporal dementia, which damages the part of the brain that controls emotions, speech, planning and judgment. Subsequent medical tests proved her right, enabling the woman to get the right support.

When Jennifer ran a care home near Bristol in the 1980s, one resident kept disappearing to a local pub where she was frequently found enjoying a pint of Guinness. Her family were horrified at her behaviour and told Jennifer it had to stop.

It turned out that the ninety-year-old woman used to be a landlady and had very much enjoyed a drink with her locals. She was reliving her younger days. Jennifer firmly believed she had undiagnosed dementia in an era when people with the condition were frequently described as 'confused'.

When Jennifer was a home care manager, her staff complained to her about a 'very difficult' elderly woman who would not let anyone past her front door. She had dementia and lived with her frail older sister.

When Jennifer called at the house, she could not get in. She spoke to the woman through the letter box and was told to go away and not trouble her any more. In speaking to the family, Jennifer discovered the woman's mother had told her as a child never to open the door to strangers.

To resolve the problem, Jennifer arranged for the carers' pictures to be put on a noticeboard in the woman's home, showing her who to expect at her home. When carers called they shouted their first name and asked her to 'check the board'. She did this and let them in every time.

Jennifer was told about the wife of an old man with dementia who was becoming difficult with carers. She criticised everything they did, saying 'this is not right' or 'you are getting it wrong'. Jennifer observed the care provided and spoke to the wife and carers.

She believed the wife was angry because she was feeling 'left out'. While having two one hour care visits each day, she was looking after her husband for the remaining twenty-two hours and did not feel valued in any way.

Jennifer advised the care workers to engage more with the wife, asking her questions, involving her in the care they provided and praising her for what she did for her husband. The change produced an immediate improvement.

These are just a few examples of the practical and emotional support Jennifer provided in working with people with dementia and carers. She helped countless numbers of people with dementia to live better, more meaningful lives.

The kind of help she offered was beneficial but frequently time consuming. In these days of fifteen-minute home care visits and care workers under pressure to make four to six home visits a day, 'troubleshooting' time is regarded as a luxury by many.

But Jennifer firmly believed that it was important to find the time to provide the right support. Helping people to live well with dementia and make the most of their abilities produced the best outcomes, and usually saved rather than cost money.

A great campaigner for better care

It's known as the 'ticking time bomb' of the twenty-first century. A condition more feared than cancer or any other illness. Something for which there is no cure and which destroys many lives.

Jennifer would talk about dementia presenting the greatest health and social care challenge to the UK over the next fifty years. She believed it would stretch every available caring and NHS resource to breaking point.

She was deeply concerned about the lack of support available for many people diagnosed with dementia, and for the small army of unpaid family carers looking after husbands, wives and parents living with the condition.

Jennifer spoke passionately at conferences and training events about the need to improve diagnosis rates, to substantially develop post-diagnostic care in local communities and raise public understanding of dementia and its consequences.

She worked hard to encourage home care providers to establish new or improved dementia care services in an era when many – particularly those working with local authorities – were experiencing budget and service cutbacks.

She played a pivotal role in improving the care of people

with dementia in their own homes, producing and delivering a ground-breaking dementia strategy for hundreds of home care providers who are members of the UKHCA.

The Skills for Care funded project was produced to deliver key elements of Prime Minister David Cameron's national 'Dementia Challenge', established to improve dementia care in England.

Published in February 2013, it became the blueprint for the UKHCA's work in helping hundreds of home care providers in England, Wales, Scotland and Northern Ireland to develop improved dementia services.

It focused on four key areas – dementia awareness and education, developing dementia-friendly communities, developing and delivering quality home care services and raising the profile of home care providers in dementia.

Jennifer planned and delivered dementia training workshops for hundreds of home care workers across the UK – from three-hour basic dementia courses to comprehensive three-day training programmes designed to challenge people's understanding of dementia.

She inspired and helped many hundreds of people who attended those UKHCA workshops, encouraging them to grow their business, develop new services and always believe in their ability to succeed.

As the dementia lead for the UKHCA, she produced a series of articles for the organisation's monthly publication, the *Homecarer*, focusing on challenging behaviour, communication, food and nutrition, and other issues.

Jennifer, in the last two years of her life, worked closely with the Social Care Institute of Excellence (SCIE) to help transform the internationally recognised online dementia information resource, the Dementia Gateway.

She defined ways to make the resource more accessible to care workers and family members caring for people with dementia. She planned and produced new content for the site focusing on early signs of dementia and diagnosis, post-diagnostic support and communication.

The new look Gateway – to which Jennifer had contributed more than any other dementia expert – was unveiled just a day after she passed away. Just a few weeks before, she took part in a filmed interview to promote the site.

She worked with the world renowned Dementia Services Development Centre (DSDC) in Stirling on a number of key projects, including editing and rewriting practical guides on food, nutrition and continence for staff caring for people with dementia.

Jennifer, an associate trainer with the DSDC for more than two years, also edited and rewrote on its behalf a major NHS Education for Scotland learning resource designed to support early interventions for people receiving a diagnosis of dementia.

Professor June Andrews, director of the DSDC, said Jennifer's work had 'significantly improved our standing, and her ability to translate mainly academic work into easily understood everyday language and her intelligent understanding of health and social care issues had proved invaluable'.

Jennifer was a consultant for Alzheimer Scotland, the country's leading dementia charity for almost three years. She spearheaded a training initiative for care staff and people from all walks of life who come into contact with people with dementia.

She worked with Stirling Council's Adult Learning Team on a ground-breaking, award-nominated Aspire training programme designed to help care workers with English as their second language look after people with dementia in residential care homes.

In 2012, she led a seven-month Alzheimer Scotland research project to assess existing post-diagnostic support for people with dementia, their families and carers in Glasgow and identify gaps and potential improvements in current services.

In the previous year, she carried out for UKHCA a major research project focusing on how to improve domiciliary care for people with dementia in the South West of England. The research was commissioned by the South West Dementia Partnership (SWDP) as part of a review of dementia services across the region.

Jennifer spoke about dementia care at national and regional conferences throughout the UK. A month before she died she was asked to help lead a dementia awareness campaign in Ghana, but had to reluctantly decline because of her failing health.

She was on the advisory board for the influential monthly publication, *The Journal of Dementia Care* and for more than a year she was an accredited trainer for the England based Jackie Pool Associates, who develop specialist dementia training programmes.

She spent many hundreds of hours talking to people with early and mid-stage dementia, including members of the Scottish Dementia Working Group, and used her wealth of experience to help others.

In 2011, Jennifer was awarded £4,000 by the Scottish Government to set up a new social enterprise to help people take holidays in dementia-friendly accommodation in a beautiful area of central Scotland.

The enterprise, Dementia Timeout, was launched after she completed a pilot project in Aberdeenshire, working with a developer to turn a bungalow in a quiet cul-de-sac into a luxury dementia-friendly holiday home.

Jennifer worked closely with Agnes Houston of the Scottish

Dementia Working Group, and a dementia champion for Scotland. Agnes stayed in the bungalow giving valuable feedback on its benefits and potential improvements.

The inspiration for Dementia Timeout came from a woman visiting the tea room Jennifer and I were working in at weekends in 2008 in Stronachlachar. She walked in with her elderly husband, ordered two coffees and sat down.

The man was staring into space. People around him seemed to be uncomfortable with this and started leaving the tea room. His wife then stood up and said: 'Please don't leave... he's not staring at you. He has dementia.'

Jennifer talked at length with her, about her difficulties in getting support, being able to go on holiday and stay in suitable accommodation and having to continually explain her husband's condition to other people.

Tributes to Jennifer's achievements were published in the UKHCA *HomeCarer* magazine, *The Journal of Dementia Care*, of which she was a member of the Advisory Board, and regional newspapers.

Mike Padgham, Chairman of UKHCA, said: 'Jennifer was a huge asset to the association from its very early days with her expert knowledge of dementia. She leaves a void that will be hard to fill and we will miss her vitality and skill.

'Her contribution to the success of the organisation over the years was tremendous. Many, many people benefited from the sharing of her knowledge and wisdom, and we owe her a great debt of gratitude for helping to make the UKHCA what it is today.

'On a personal level, I always found Jennifer a charming, warm and friendly person dedicated to improving the care of others and to making a very real difference to the lives of those with dementia.'

Bridget Warr, Chief Executive of the UKHCA, said Jennifer 'believed passionately that caring for those with dementia was the greatest challenge facing social care today.

'Jennifer brought huge warmth, competence and expertise to the association in all her work and was well respected throughout the home care sector in the UK. We are feeling her loss keenly.'

Lucianne Sawyer, President of UKHCA, said 'promoting quality was very much Jennifer's driving force as was shown so clearly in her very lively and enjoyable training sessions, which were such a feature of her work with members, and for which she will be greatly missed.

'It is the lively enthusiasm and lasting friendship which has endeared her to all those of us who were fortunate enough to encounter or work with her, and certainly what I am going to miss most.

'I particularly admire the work she has done on dementia, which has ensured that we are regarded as serious participants in trying to ensure that home care providers are able to provide an appropriate and competent service.'

The SCIE's Joanne Lenham, who worked with Jennifer on the Dementia Gateway, said 'Jennifer was an absolute delight to work with and made such a huge contribution to various aspects of my work over the last couple of years. I really valued her knowledge and expertise, and her ability to understand just what we needed, and how she delivered it to such a high standard.'

Catherine Ross, editor of *The Journal of Dementia Care*, said Jennifer was 'a woman with many skills and had so much to offer the field of dementia care, and she will be greatly missed.'

The future and unfinished business

How do we defuse the dementia ticking time bomb? How will we cope with increasing numbers of people with dementia at a time when our health and social care services are being stretched to the limit?

How do we ease the pressure on the hundreds of thousands of unpaid carers providing twenty-four-hour-a-day care for aged parents, brothers, sisters and friends living with dementia in their own homes?

Governments and health chiefs throughout the UK have launched new initiatives to substantially increase diagnosis rates and the level of post-diagnostic and palliative support in communities.

Dozens of dementia-friendly cities, towns and villages are being established across England, Scotland, Wales and Northern Ireland to co-ordinate and provide improved care and support for people with dementia and their carers.

Jennifer had a simple formula for tackling the challenges ahead:

*The key is providing the right advice, care and support
at the right time from pre-diagnosis to end stage dementia,*

113

and helping people with dementia to live well with
dementia by enabling them to make the most of their
abilities.

We need many more experienced and well trained
dementia advisers, nurses and care staff in our
communities, in care homes and in hospitals to provide the
high calibre care and support required.

And we must offer greater help to the army of unpaid
family carers who look after relatives with dementia twenty-
four hours a day, seven days a week. Without them, our
health and social care services would collapse.

Our whole approach to dementia has to be pro-active,
not reactive. It can't be crisis-led as it is in many cases
today. There is clear evidence that a change is happening...
but we have a long, long way to go.

She knew it would take a 'monumental effort' to make this
happen. But she warned that the alternative was 'a growing
crisis that will not only crush our health and social care services
but destroy more and more families'.

Jennifer left no-one in any doubt about the enormity of the
task facing governments, the NHS and social care in providing
essential support and care for people with dementia and their
carers.

In a detailed briefing note to a large company looking to
take her on as a consultant, and written just two weeks before
she passed away, she made the following observations about the
state of dementia care in the UK.

There is so much to do and so little time to achieve
what needs to be done. Throwing more and more money at
dementia is not necessarily the solution. We have to make

sure the money already available is spent in the best possible way – to help people with dementia live meaningful, fulfilling lives and make the most of their abilities. Sadly, enormous amounts of money are still being spent on caring for people with dementia in hospital when many don't need to be there. That money would be better invested in keeping them well at home or in care homes where proper care is provided.

Dementia diagnosis is a lottery across the UK – good in Scotland and parts of Northern Ireland but generally poor elsewhere. Why? Partly because some GPs are not convinced it is a good idea to tell someone they may have dementia when there are no post-diagnostic services in place to support them. Partly because some people do not want the diagnosis because of the impact it will have on their lives. And partly because there are too few resources – educational, medical and financial – in place to ensure the help required is effective. Hundreds of thousands believed to have dementia have not been diagnosed and have little or no access to professional help.

Many local authority financed home care services are still time and task focused and are not geared to offering person-centred care, or what someone really wants. Across the UK the vast majority of these services are only available to people who are in critical need, and most people with dementia do not qualify for help. More and more is being expected of unpaid family carers to provide care 24/7, many of whom have little or no support. New initiatives are being developed to help cope with the looming dementia crisis, but there is justification in the argument that Government and NHS intervention, particularly in England and Wales, is 'too little too late'. Scotland is the only country providing anything like comprehensive help for people with dementia and their families from the point of diagnosis to receiving individual, person-centred post-diagnostic support. But hospital care throughout the UK for people with dementia is still, in too many cases, way below the standard it should be.

There are, of course, many examples of good dementia care in the home care and care home sectors. Best practice is being shared and at long last different organisations are talking to each other about the way forward and sharing knowledge. Dementia-friendly cities, towns and villages are springing up all over the UK and it is up to all of us with good experience in dementia care and with the will to make things better to take up the challenge of making these important initiatives work and thrive. This is not the time to stand back and see what happens. Everyone who can make a positive contribution must become involved for all our sakes.

Jennifer firmly believed that dementia training had to be delivered in different ways to suit different situations. She devised and delivered innovative new training programmes for eye care specialists and dentists to improve care for people with dementia.

She worked closely with opticians and dentists to show how day-to-day practices, eye and dental check-ups and their premises could be made more dementia-friendly. Her ideas were pioneered in the UK, setting the benchmark for training in these fields.

She spent many hours in eye and dental clinics to observe how tests are carried out and how they could be improved. She demonstrated the benefits of better communication and involving carers in eye and dental tests.

Jennifer was about to put together new dementia focused training programmes for doctors' surgeries, shops, restaurants and cafes, supermarkets and airports, and bus and train stations when she passed away.

She was concerned that many organisations believed their staff were 'dementia savvy' after a basic three-hour course designed to provide a minimal understanding of dementia and the behaviour of people with the condition.

'Training has to be ongoing for us all. No two people experience dementia in the same way, so we are learning new ways of helping people all the time. It's vital that good support and outcomes are shared for everyone's benefit,' she said.

In late 2013, Jennifer took part in Alzheimer's Society research into future training requirements for home care. 'This is a really positive initiative and I expect great things of it,' she said.

Jennifer believed that, as the number of people with dementia increased, more and more family carers would learn from their own experience rather than through receiving 'not always available' professional help.

'Twenty years ago everyone knew someone with cancer and gained knowledge about certain symptoms and behaviour. Today, virtually everyone knows someone with dementia and there are many people providing all the care without expert help.

'Many turn to forums, such as Alzheimer's Society's Talking Point, to discuss their worries. We have to learn from this, understand the real issues affecting people every day and use them as a platform to provide better care and support,' she said.

Jennifer believed it was critical for all of us – from primary school children to businesses, public transport, leisure and sports employees and shop and hotel workers – to have an understanding of dementia and how to help someone with it.

She was a great advocate of early diagnosis of dementia,

regardless of age. Because it was the only way of ensuring the person with dementia received the right advice, help and support at the right time.

But she frequently warned that unless there were sufficient post-diagnostic support services in place, people showing early symptoms of dementia would become increasingly reluctant to seek a diagnosis.

'Many who are working, driving and with family commitments – particularly those with early onset dementia – will avoid getting a diagnosis if there are no support structures in place. Because they fear they will lose everything and no-one will be there to help them,' she said.

Jennifer said everyone in society had a role to play in removing the stigma experienced by some people with dementia and understanding the potentially devastating impact the condition had on those with the condition and their families.

'Many people with dementia will go on to lose their driving licence, their jobs and their ability to work. They will need considerable help in adjusting to a new life, in getting the right advice and support in going forward.

'Insurance companies, banks and others will have to be encouraged to take a positive approach in these circumstances, and not look to make life even more challenging for people diagnosed with dementia.

'It is also important to remember that many people caring for loved ones with dementia have to give up their work and social activities to provide 24/7 support. The cost to them is huge and they have to bear the financial burden themselves.'

As dementia lead for the UKHCA, Jennifer campaigned vigorously for home care staff to have a greater voice and influence in the care and support of people living with dementia in their own homes.

While carrying out a major research project for the organisation, she identified home care as the 'poor relation' in providing continuing assistance for people with dementia and family carers.

She discovered home care staff were frequently not consulted by GPs, nurses and social care professionals diagnosing and monitoring changes in people with dementia even though they spent the greatest amount of time with the people involved and their families.

'They have so much information that is useful in making a diagnosis or planning care, from being in the home and observing a person's behaviour on a day-to-day basis, yet they are often overlooked by professionals,' she said.

This is changing, with more home care providers being involved in 'multi-agency' consultations on care and support planning. But Jennifer predicted it would take 'many long years' for home care to get the recognition it deserved.

She was a great campaigner for better, person-centred care allowing people with dementia and their families to make their own decisions on what support they needed, be it with a hobby, going shopping or personal care.

She believed that people with dementia and their families should be given greater control of any funding provided for their care. This is happening, through direct payments and 'personal budgets', but the change was far too gradual for Jennifer's liking.

Her work on the UKHCA Dementia Strategy included developing important new links to connect home care providers to businesses and other organisations in dementia-friendly communities.

The task was far from finished when she passed away. But she played a significant role in encouraging providers to support and take part in national dementia awareness weeks organised by the Alzheimer's Association and Alzheimer Scotland.

In helping to encourage providers to develop and deliver quality dementia services, Jennifer established a number of focus groups on LinkedIn with a view to creating a nationwide online support network.

She sought and received examples of good practice in dementia care and these were published on the UKHCA website. But she acknowledged that making this an effective resource would 'take some considerable time to achieve'.

Unlike the voluntary sector, she found home care reluctant to engage with social media. 'Much more has to be done to educate providers on the benefits of using LinkedIn, Twitter and Facebook if real progress is to be made,' she said.

4.

Life after
Jennifer's
passing

It was the saddest and hardest walk I have ever had to make. But I was doing it for a good reason, to fulfil one of Jennifer's last wishes. And I was not alone. Jennifer's brother, Stephen, stood shoulder to shoulder with me as I made my way through the heart of Stirling city centre.

I was delivering the last item of clothing she would wear on this earth – her wedding dress – to the undertaker's in Baker Street. It was a genuinely surreal moment, something I could never have imagined doing, something I would never have wanted to carry out.

Jennifer had worn the beautiful ivory gown twice before, when we married at Dundas Castle in March 2003 and at the special service to bless our wedding in Charmouth.

I found it packed away in a box at home. The night before I took it to Stirling, I laid it out on our bed. I then watched Stephen spend several hours gently cleaning away marks on the dress to ensure it looked perfect for a two-day celebration of Jennifer's life.

My emotions were running high as we arrived at the car park at the Marches Shopping Centre in Stirling, and began the ten-minute walk to the undertaker's through the indoor shopping centre to Port Street, King's Street and then on to Baker Street.

No-one would have known I was carrying a wedding dress. It was in a white plastic cover which I held so tightly to my chest. I was oblivious to the hundreds of shoppers I walked past on my journey. I could only think of the previous happy occasions I had seen Jennifer in the dress.

I was in tears when I arrived at the offices of Somers and Currid. But it was at that point that a huge emotional weight was lifted from my shoulders. For the first time, I realised I had done something positive, something Jennifer would have been proud of.

Celebrating Jennifer's life turned into a very personal tribute, reflecting key events in our lives, from when we became engaged in Somerset in 2001 to our wedding and the renewal of our vows in Lanzarote on our tenth wedding anniversary.

A piper played traditional Scottish music as people arrived at the historic and picturesque church at the gateway to the Trossachs. Jennifer's brother and I were wearing full Highland dress – Flower of Scotland tartan kilts, Bonnie Prince Charlie jackets and waistcoats and sgian-dubhs in our kilt hose.

The sun was shining and the snow-covered Ben Lomond

Mountain could be seen in all its glory from the steps leading up to the church. At first glance, passers-by would have guessed that they were seeing the beginning of a wedding ceremony.

The celebration was taking place at St Mary's Church, above the main street of Aberfoyle, thirteen days after she passed away. The tartan Stephen and I were dressed in was identical to that worn at my wedding more than ten years earlier.

Music played during the service was from our wedding, from Libera's rousing *Jubilate* to haunting and beautiful music from the Oscar winning movie *Braveheart*. One of the readings, *Two pebbles, two hearts – our love story*, was composed by myself in 2003 and first read at our marriage ceremony.

The piece from *Braveheart* was particularly moving as it was played when Jennifer walked down the aisle towards me on the happiest day of our lives. It included the haunting music that marked the highly emotional point at which William Wallace and his wife were 'reunited in death'.

I wore the Dalvey pocket watch Jennifer had given me on our wedding day. Stephen wore the thistle brooch I had given to Jennifer purchased from Edinburgh's Luckenbooth shop. My son, David, wore Saltire cufflinks I had adorned at Dundas.

Two large wedding pictures given pride of place in our home were displayed in the church along with a memorable photograph of Jennifer above a golden beach on the Isle of Harris. This was not a farewell or a funeral, but an intimate expression of admiration and adoration for a truly remarkable woman and wife.

Jennifer had never been to the tiny church, so intricate, so intimate, so beautiful, but that didn't matter... it was absolutely the right place for the occasion. Family, friends and professional colleagues travelled from as far afield as New Zealand, Holland, Switzerland and Cornwall to be there.

The rector, Richard Grosse, played a pivotal role, reciting *Two pebbles, two hearts – our love story* and other readings. Stephen recited my tribute to Jennifer and the following day, at a family-only cremation service, read his own personal accolade (published at the end of this section).

Songs played at the cremation service included Louis Armstrong's 'What a Wonderful World', which Jennifer played every time she had dialysis, Barbra Streisand's 'Evergreen', probably Jennifer's all-time favourite, and Luther Vandross and Mariah Carey's version of 'My Endless Love', which we played on our tenth wedding anniversary.

The 'wake' or get-together to continue the celebration of Jennifer's life was held at the idyllic Roman Camp Hotel in Callander. Again, it was a place she had never visited, but she would have loved its calm and elegant ambience. Collections for Macmillan Cancer Support and the British Kidney Patient Association raised almost £1,000.

When Jennifer's ashes were ready for collection I took the same walk I had made with her wedding dress, but in reverse, and this time with my son, David. We stepped slowly and silently out into Stirling's Baker Street, down King's Street and through the main shopping centre.

I hugged the urn containing Jennifer's ashes close to my chest. As I was about to get into a lift to take me to the car park, a woman security guard smiled at me and said: 'You must be carrying something very precious to be holding it so close.' She was right, although she couldn't know what it was.

Just under four months later, a beautiful oak bench crafted in memory of Jennifer was unveiled at Stronachlachar on the banks of Loch Katrine. Made by Gartmore carpenter Tom Percival from a 300-year-old oak tree felled in storms in Scotland in 2011, it is a genuine work of art.

It was put in place on March 17, 2014, St Patrick's Day, and the date of Jennifer's baptism in Wells, Somerset in 1963.

The bench is in one of the most beautiful, calm and peaceful spots in central Scotland, overlooking the hills and loch we loved. It is just a few yards from the holiday cottage where we first stayed and fell in love with this tiny community in 2006.

I am delighted to say that Jennifer's bench is now one of the most sat on, most admired and most photographed benches in Scotland. It is a fitting and lasting memorial to her – a reminder of the great things she achieved, her kindness and never-say-die attitude.

A second memorial bench has been placed in the grounds of the Bishop's Palace in Wells by Jennifer's parents. Again, it is in an idyllic spot so enjoyed by Jennifer as she grew up in the historic city.

The day my whole world stopped

How do you begin to build a new life after losing the person you most cherish – the woman who became my soulmate, my greatest friend and who was at the very core of everything wonderful in my existence?

It's a good question and one I have no answer to. I am still unable to imagine a worthwhile future without Jennifer. My whole world stopped when she passed away and I don't know how or when it will start again.

It often feels I am in a kind of suspended animation – sometimes struggling to survive from day-to-day, unable to plan ahead and caught up in an alternative universe where everyone else is getting on with their lives.

I miss Jennifer more than words could ever say. I feel so alone and lost without her, frequently hopeless and crave the love, passion, hugs, kisses, smiles, warmth and almost telepathic understanding we shared.

At the same time, I am uplifted by the many good memories of our precious time together. I know how fortunate I was to meet and marry Jennifer, and to enjoy such a rare and beautiful relationship.

The inevitable clash of feelings results in good and bad days, vulnerable times when I want to lock myself away from everyone else and moments when a kind word or gesture gives me renewed hope.

We all experience the death of someone close in different ways. There is no pattern of feelings or behaviour. No correct way of doing or not doing something. No simple way to explain what is unfolding.

Important birthdays and anniversaries are immensely challenging. I experience my darkest times between the fourth and ninth days of each month. It was on those six days in November 2013 that Jennifer was taken to and ultimately passed away in hospital.

I relive every moment of her time in intensive care: her struggles to stay alive, to overcome the greatest crisis in her life; the sleepless nights, the raw heartache, the fear of losing my Jennifer.

Perhaps the pain of those six days will ease with time. Perhaps the flashbacks will become less regular. But, for the time being, they remain a traumatic and graphic reminder of the worst period of my life.

It has been important for me to stay 'close' to Jennifer through surrounding myself with pictures of holidays and important milestones in our life... our first meeting, our engagement, wedding day and wedding anniversaries.

I had her wedding ring enlarged to enable me to wear it next to my wedding ring. I purchased a chain to wear her engagement and other special rings around my neck... and close to my heart.

I started to carry with me everywhere the first picture of Jennifer and me, taken when we attended a family barbecue in Devon. The photo was one of two she had by her bedside in hospital when she fell ill.

Framed words we had written or chosen for each other gained increased significance. I displayed them on bedroom cabinets, window sills and tables, reading them with great affection each day.

I constantly read and re-read cards and love letters we had sent to each other – stored in boxes and bags throughout the house – and listened to music that had featured so strongly in our lives together.

I found great comfort in Eva Cassidy's versions of 'Songbird', 'Autumn Leaves', 'Time After Time' and 'Over the Rainbow'. The haunting words seemed so relevant, so powerful, as I grieved.

The songs of Barbra Streisand and Celine Dion, Jennifer's favourite singers, and moving passages from books and poems we both treasured, proved so uplifting at the most difficult times.

I looked at the film of our wedding time and time again, reliving the happiest day of our lives, and watched endless hours of funny and memorable videos we had made in the last year of Jennifer's life.

I craved calm and peace, finding it time and time again at St Mary's Church in Aberfoyle and at the Roman Camp Hotel in Callander, where the celebration of Jennifer's life had taken place.

I experienced great tranquillity in our garden in Stronachlachar, particularly as spring arrived in 2014 after one of the wettest winters in history, new blooms bringing much needed colour to the rockery and to my life.

I also found peace on Jennifer's memorial bench overlooking Loch Katrine, sitting there in all weathers for endless hours day after day, watching the sun set and rise and brilliant full moons.

Amid the devastation I was feeling, all these 'coping

mechanisms' helped me to find reasons to keep going, to avoid continuously collapsing in tears, and to remember the joy we had brought to each other.

I still gain enormous comfort from seeing and hearing Jennifer in our videos, looking at her amazing smile in our pictures, reading our love letters and cards and sitting in our garden and on 'Jenny's bench', which I can see from my home.

I am always talking out loud to Jennifer, chatting away at home and on my travels about everyday happenings, my fears, how much I love and miss her and recollecting all the good times we had.

Reading everything from *Lord of the Rings* and George RR Martin's *Song of Ice and Fire* series to Conn Iggulden's take on the *War of the Roses*, has provided a great escape from the harsh realities of day-to-day life.

Visiting places we loved has become a real tonic, particularly Jennifer's favourite view (Loch Arklet and the Arrochar Alps), Inveraray, St Andrews, Skye and the awe-inspiring mountains of Glencoe and the Cairngorms.

Holidays, though, are a step too far. As are eating out and going to the cinema and theatre alone. I value the sanctuary of home. It is my key to coping, where I feel closest of all to Jennifer.

So far, I have decided against seeking 'official' bereavement counselling. I was taught from a young age that the only way to tackle a crisis is to 'face it head on and deal with it yourself'. Good advice or not, it has worked for me many times.

I know I can't get through this alone. I talk to two to three good friends, my son and Jennifer's family whose advice and support has proved invaluable. They are always 'there for me' when I need them and have never let me down.

Securing part-time work at the now Pier Cafe in

Stronachlachar helped to give me fresh purpose and value and to face the many challenges of living alone, looking after the house – and myself.

Nothing and no-one though can fill the huge hole Jennifer has left behind. The pain of losing her regularly feels as raw as the day she passed away. But her determination to never give up hope and to stay positive will live on in me.

A trip down memory lane

The beach was deserted. I had walked along the promenade at Burnham-on-Sea for an hour or so before stepping out onto the vast stretch of sand, carrying a small grey rounded stone in my right hand.

I was retracing steps Jennifer had taken more than thirteen years earlier when she threw a pebble into the sea while making a wish to find true love – just as I was doing the same thing on a Scottish island.

I was completely inappropriately dressed for the windy weather and for walking on the beach. I had my best leather shoes and trousers on, and a thin, short-sleeved shirt.

It was low tide and I faced a long walk to reach the sea. I stupidly ignored warnings displayed on the promenade about the sinking sand and found myself trudging slowly and aimlessly through a mud 'soup'.

My shoes disappeared into a thick brown sludge. I just about managed to pull myself out, falling over spectacularly in the process, but hanging on grimly to the pebble, determined to follow in Jennifer's footsteps.

I found a safer route, closer to the sea. I took aim, threw the stone and missed the target. I picked up another pebble, inched a little closer to the low water mark, tried again and this time hit the water.

I had three different wishes – for the strength to cope with a life without her, for our love to last for eternity and to be reunited with Jennifer after my death.

Jennifer would have laughed out loud at me getting stuck in the mud, falling over and struggling to reach the sea. Anyone witnessing my spontaneous antics would have thought I was drunk or mad.

But I had no regrets about doing what I did. It lifted my spirits, made me smile and gave me the opportunity to relive a moment that had transformed our lives all those years ago.

It was March 2014, four months after Jennifer's passing, and I had travelled to Somerset to spend time with her family before heading for Cornwall to stay with friends.

I had not planned to go to Burnham. I had been to Exeter to see a friend and was on my way to Jennifer's parents' home in Wells when I suddenly decided to head further north on the M5.

I drove to the house Jennifer and I first lived in, in Burnham's Pinter Close, walked down the high street and visited the local Tesco store where I bought flowers for her on our second date in early 2001.

Memories of so many good times together came flooding back. The weather was terrible, cold, wet and very windy, but it didn't matter a jot. It was an off-the-wall day I will never forget.

My trip south was the first time I had been away from home since Jennifer passed away. Family and friends had encouraged me to make the journey. It gave me a real boost at the right time.

I enjoyed the silence and peace in Wells Cathedral and

walked by the moat outside the city's Bishop's Palace – two things Jennifer and I enjoyed doing when we visited her parents and other relatives.

I watched a home game for Wells RFC, rekindling my passion for watching live rugby matches. I walked for miles along the city's cobbled streets, just as Jennifer had done in her childhood and teenage years.

With Jennifer's mother, I attended a Sunday morning service at St Cuthbert's Church, listening to the choir in which Jennifer had once been a key figure and appreciated the building's almost cathedral-like architecture.

Some of the choristers she sang with back in the 1970s and early 80s were still there, and in the congregation were a number of people who remembered her with great fondness and admiration.

The last time I had been there was with Jennifer in November 2012 to attend the annual Remembrance Day service and parade in which she had featured year after year in her younger days.

My time in Somerset gave me the confidence to get out and about on my own, to spend valuable time with her family. It also gave me the opportunity to discover more about Jennifer's early days and favourite childhood haunts.

Most importantly, it encouraged me to write this book, to tell Jennifer's story, to enable people to read about her remarkable life and to be enthused and moved by what she achieved in her fifty-one years.

I didn't want her accomplishments, her compelling story, to die with her. I wanted to shout from the rooftops about her and what she had done in her life. I very much hope this tribute to her achieves this.

The enormous power of the human spirit and to do good

has been illustrated in the life and death of Stephen Sutton, the Staffordshire teenager who died of colorectal cancer in May 2014.

He raised more than £4 million for the Teenage Cancer Trust and inspired millions with his positive attitude. Jennifer and Stephen had so much in common, particularly a determination to triumph against the greatest of odds.

We can all learn so much from both of them.

The final word goes to Muriel Laity, my 'adopted' mother in Cornwall, who looked after me when I got my first job as a trainee reporter in the 1970s. She met Jennifer just a few times and was thrilled when we attended her surprise eightieth birthday party in May 2013.

Muriel, who has met thousands of people in her time, in her home village of Crowlas, near Penzance in Cornwall and through holidays and the church, said: 'Jennifer was the loveliest and bravest woman I have ever known.'

5.

Stephen's tribute to Jennifer: my big sister

Read at the celebration of her life in Scotland in November 2013.

Where do I start? Jennifer is such a positive soul, a larger than life character, who touched so many people's lives in such deep and meaningful ways. Jennifer is one of those rare, exceptional people who always thought of others before herself, how to help, how to support, how to guide and how to protect. She never saw the bad in people and always looked at life as a glass half full. There was always a way forward and always a route to a better place.

Jennifer trained as a nurse, a caring, giving and compassionate career that mirrored her and complemented her character and personality perfectly. She learned her trade from lecturers, doctors and consultants, working hard, caring for others. Even while suffering from kidney failure Jennifer continued to work, determined to be judged on her efforts and merit rather than accept any concessions because of her illness. That dogged determination and indomitable personality continued to propel her throughout her life.

When she moved into the dementia arena she became one of the pre-eminent dementia care specialists. In true Jennifer style she looked at the situation, spotted where people needed help, and devised a plan to link all aspects of dementia care into a cohesive strategy and framework.

Jennifer recently celebrated twenty-nine years with Fred, her transplanted kidney, astounding and amazing all the experts. Even when faced with her most recent challenge, inoperable, terminal lung cancer she continued to ignore and confound all the medical experts, surviving a full twelve months post-diagnosis and achieving, with Paul's unswerving love, help and support, true quality of life.

Throughout my entire life, from good times to bad, from the dizzy peaks of success and happiness to the darkest depths of despair, I have always known that I had a guardian angel with me. Someone to turn to, someone to support me; never judgmental, always positive, always supportive. Whatever the season, day of the week, time of the day or issues in her life I had this unmistakable truth and comfort; that there was someone there for me, watching out for me, picking me up and dusting me off, even when all others had melted away... my big sister.

Jennifer had the great fortune to meet Paul twelve years ago and fall deeply in love. I have watched, with admiration and happiness, their relationship and love, blossom and grow. When Jennifer and Paul married in 2003 she offered me the great honour and privilege to be the person to give her away at her wedding. An offer I humbly accepted, and it proved to be, without doubt the proudest moment of my life. For I knew, that day, I was giving my sister away to a man that would love her as much as she loved him. Who would always put her first and be there for her, just as she had always been there for everyone else. My big sister had found true happiness, tranquillity, an equal and a soulmate.

We all know that Jennifer was a deeply spiritual person with a strong belief that events were never a coincidence; there was always a plan.

On November 9, 2013 some might say Jennifer lost her fight with cancer. I prefer to believe that her loved ones from the spirit world took her into their care to prevent her, and us suffering; indeed Jennifer probably had a hand in this, once again thinking of all of us first.

My sister simply did not know how to lose. She lived by the mantra 'live every day as if it's your last, because one day you'll be right'. She lived life to the full and like warm summer sunshine brightened up every life she touched, always smiling, always caring, always with time to spare.

I have spent the last few difficult days informing people of Jennifer's passing. I have been truly humbled by the sheer volume and intensity of praise and admiration for my big sister. So many people have found Jennifer to be a hugely important person, of great kindness and compassion, in their lives.

There is a saying, which is often lightly used: 'they broke the mould when they made this one'. Well, I can tell you, that whichever mould they used to make Jennifer it was sensational, and she did not just break the mould she vaporised it. My sister was an inspirational person, loving, *talented, supportive, compassionate and wise beyond her years. A truly wonderful and unique human being, who will never be forgotten by anyone who had the good fortune to know her.*

During her all too short time with us she burned brighter and stronger than the brightest of stars in the heavens. I would say I consider myself lucky to have known the amazing, inspirational, force of nature that is Jennifer. But to have been gifted Jennifer as my sister... I would have to say I have been blessed beyond imagination. Never has one person given so much, to so many, so freely, unconditionally and with such regularity.

Since Jennifer passed over there is now a huge hole in mine and all our lives. But I have no doubts, in true Jennifer style, we will not have heard the last of her. For Jennifer, my outstanding, amazing, inspirational and brilliant sister, rules, opinions and conventional wisdom were just simply there to be proved wrong.